Pregnancy
& Diabetes

A COMPLETE
GUIDE FOR WOMEN
WITH GESTATIONAL,
TYPE 2, AND TYPE 1
DIABETES

Marina Chaparro,
RD, CDE, MPH

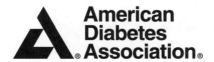

Director, Book Operations, Victor Van Beuren; *Managing Editor, Books,* John Clark; *Associate Director, Book Marketing,* Annette Reape; *Acquisitions Editor,* Jaclyn Konich; *Copyeditor,* Brian Keating; *Composition,* Circle Graphics; *Cover Design,* Vis-à-vis Creative; *Printer,* Versa Press.

Printed in the United States of America

1 3 5 7 9 10 8 6 4 2

The suggestions and information contained in this publication are generally consistent with the *Standards of Medical Care in Diabetes* and other policies of the American Diabetes Association, but they do not represent the policy or position of the Association or any of its boards or committees. Reasonable steps have been taken to ensure the accuracy of the information presented. However, the American Diabetes Association cannot ensure the safety or efficacy of any product or service described in this publication. Individuals are advised to consult a physician or other appropriate healthcare professional before undertaking any diet or exercise program or taking any medication referred to in this publication. Professionals must use and apply their own professional judgment, experience, and training and should not rely solely on the information contained in this publication before prescribing any diet, exercise, or medication. The American Diabetes Association—its officers, directors, employees, volunteers, and members—assumes no responsibility or liability for personal or other injury, loss, or damage that may result from the suggestions or information in this publication.

Mindy Saraco conducted the internal review of this book to ensure that it meets American Diabetes Association guidelines.

♾ The paper in this publication meets the requirements of the ANSI Standard Z39.48-1992 (permanence of paper).

ADA titles may be purchased for business or promotional use or for special sales. To purchase more than 50 copies of this book at a discount, or for custom editions of this book with your logo, contact the American Diabetes Association at the address below or at booksales@diabetes.org.

American Diabetes Association

2451 Crystal Drive, Suite 900

Arlington, VA 22202

DOI: 10.2337/9781580407304

Library of Congress Control Number: 2020942629

CONTENTS

PREGNANCY & DIABETES ACKNOWLEDGMENTS

Never did I imagine nineteen years ago, lying in that hospital bed after being diagnosed with type 1 diabetes, that I would be writing this story of love, dedication, and hard work! This book is my gift to every brave woman with diabetes who is about to embark on this journey. Know that you can do this!

To my parents: Thank you for giving me the greatest gift I could ask for: Never allowing me to give up on my dreams. Your love, support, and example have made me who I am today.

To my sisters, my biggest cheerleaders in life, thank you for your endless love and for never complaining when you had to eat sugar-free cookies.

Thank you to my amazing colleagues, diabetes educators, contributors, and my healthcare team, for their invaluable advice and support. Thank you for believing in this crazy idea!

To my Husband, *my Morrito*, I couldn't have asked for a better partner in life. You held my hand when I needed it the most and continue to do so every single day.

Dedicated to my daughters, Emma Lucia and Alicia. You are my source of inspiration. Your births have been the most challenging and rewarding thing I've done in my life: It was all worth it!

INTRODUCTION

What to Expect in
Pregnancy & Diabetes

You got this, mama!

Diabetes in pregnancy can be stressful, scary, and filled with doubts. *"Can I have a healthy pregnancy if I have diabetes?" "What can I eat?" "How do I keep my blood glucose in target?" "Why me?" "Will my baby be okay?"* Whether you have been diagnosed with gestational diabetes, live with type 2 diabetes, or have been living with type 1 diabetes since age 5, diabetes during pregnancy can make you feel alone and overwhelmed. But trust me, you are not alone. These 9 months of pregnancy can and will be filled with health and happiness. With the right tools, careful planning, and support, you will be able to have a successful pregnancy.

Research shows that women with diabetes who receive pre-conception planning and who are well managed before and during pregnancy reduce their risks of developing complications to about the same rates as women who don't have diabetes. Maintaining blood glucose as close to normal as possible will be critical in the next 9 months and is beneficial even before becoming pregnant. Fortunately, this book will show you how to get there! Checking blood glucose seven or more times a day, having to inject insulin, seeing doctors multiple times, measuring foods, reading labels, and counting carbohydrates—it's all part of this journey. Whether you are new to the diabetes journey or have been doing it a long time, know this: you are not alone, and you can have a healthy pregnancy. Diabetes management during pregnancy may be demanding, but it's also so worth it!

Pregnancy & Diabetes is a book that will guide, teach, and empower pregnant women with diabetes to enjoy a healthy and beautiful pregnancy. This book gives moms-to-be practical and easy-to-follow advice on how to successfully manage diabetes during the 9 months of pregnancy. This book is for the woman with gestational, type 2, or type 1 diabetes who is planning for or going through pregnancy and who wants everyday solutions to the unique challenges that arise during pregnancy with diabetes.

Diabetes in pregnancy is a very personal subject for me. I was diagnosed with type 1 diabetes when I was 16 years old. The diagnosis shaped my life and, subsequently, my decision to pursue nutritional sciences. I studied nutrition because I was personally affected by a chronic condition that was deeply rooted in what I ate. But more important, I wanted to empower others living with diabetes to lead a healthy and happy life. For the past 12 years, I've worked at leading diabetes institutions helping families, women, and children with diabetes *thrive*. I had thought that with this extensive background in diabetes management and nutritional science, diabetes in pregnancy would be an easy subject for me, but boy was I wrong!

Managing diabetes in pregnancy was no easy task. There were many days of frustration and worry, but it was all worth it, and it's been my biggest reward in life. After having two healthy pregnancies with diabetes, I can tell you that having a healthy and happy pregnancy is possible. This is the reason I am writing this book. Not only do I have the professional experience and training, but I understand firsthand the daily struggles of this journey. It is my way of giving back. This book was created to give you the tools, strategies, and motivation to keep going even when you think you can't, all inspired by the things I wish someone had told me before and during my pregnancy.

This book has been a journey of love, dedication, and passion. Without realizing it, this book began before my first daughter was born. Before my pregnancy, I did a lot of research on this topic, spoke to experts in the field, and looked for support groups where I could get information. I had a hard time finding information that was practical and relatable, and not focused on the clinical aspects. While other books on pregnancy and diabetes offer a one-size-fits-all approach by treating gestational, type 2, and type 1 diabetes the same, this book gives unique, simple, and to-the-point recommendations for each audience based on their specific needs.

If you have been looking for a resource to help you navigate the ins and outs of pregnancy with diabetes, this book is for you. This book will provide real advice with everyday scenarios that will teach you *how* to manage your diabetes in the 9 months of your pregnancy. My goal is to translate the latest scientific research on diabetes and pregnancy into practical insights and pearls of wisdom you could easily apply to your day-to-day life. You will find answers to many of your frequent questions, get meal plan and snack ideas and review the latest technology in diabetes care during pregnancy. *Pregnancy & Diabetes* is a valuable guide that will teach you how to successfully manage your diabetes during pregnancy without sacrificing the love and joy this experience brings.

When I was diagnosed with diabetes, I remember receiving my first diabetes book edited by the American Diabetes Association. It changed my life. Fast-forward to 20 years after my diagnosis, and here I am, writing this book. It has been my life's mission to help people with diabetes lead a healthy and balanced life. I became a diabetes educator and registered dietitian because of my diagnosis, and I've worked with hundreds of people with diabetes. But most important, I've *lived* through two healthy pregnancies with diabetes. I hope this book changes your life, changes your pregnancy, and empowers you to lead a healthy pregnancy.

Marina Chaparro, RD, CDE, MPH
Mom, Registered Dietitian and Diabetes Educator
Founder of GoodLife Diabetes & Nutrichicos
Find out more at www.goodlifediabetes.com

HOW TO USE
THIS BOOK

This book is separated into four sections: "Gestational Diabetes and Pregnancy," "Type 2 Diabetes and Pregnancy," "Type 1 Diabetes and Pregnancy," and "Resources for All." If you're wondering why this book separated into three different types of diabetes, the answer is simple: Not all pregnancies with diabetes are alike. Yes, they do share similarities, but they should not be treated with a one-size-fits-all approach. When I was pregnant with my first daughter, I was frustrated when I would get a book on diabetes and pregnancy, and come to find out it didn't mention any information that was relevant to what I was experiencing. This separation allows for more in-depth coverage of the specific aspects unique to each type of diabetes. In each of the first three sections, you will find insights specific to each condition, while the last section, "Resources for All," is meant to cover information and strategies helpful to *all* pregnant women, regardless of the type of diabetes. This by no means should limit you from reading the book in its entirety, as I am sure you will find useful takeaways in each section. In the "Resources for All" section, you will find useful resources such as snack ideas, meal plans with tasty and simple recipes, a Q&A section, and information on apps, technology, and stress management. This is by far my favorite section, so make sure to read it all! Throughout this book, you will find real advice by women who have gone through pregnancy and know first-hand what it was like to go through this experience. I believe that sharing real advice is sometimes more powerful because it conveys the reality of living through the successes and throughout the pregnancy journey.

You will find recommended chapters in each of the introductory sections to make it easy for you to navigate and get the most out of this book. If you have gestational diabetes, I encourage you to first read that section, followed by "Resources for All." You might also benefit from reading the "Type 2 Diabetes" section as they share some similarities. If you have type 2 diabetes, I encourage you to first read that section, followed by "Resources for All." Many people with type 2 diabetes are on medication, but if you are not, I recommend you read section 1 (Gestational Diabetes), where you'll find information that can apply to you. If you are on medications like insulin, or even using a pump, read along into section 3 (Type 1 Diabetes), where you might find relevant information on technology and what to expect in each trimester.

This book is easy to read, and you can find a wealth of information by reviewing all the sections. In the end, all pregnant women with diabetes share one common goal: having a healthy baby!

SECTION

1

Gestational Diabetes and Pregnancy

SECTION 1
Gestational Diabetes and Pregnancy

Recommended Chapters to Review

- Chapter 9: Managing Blood Glucose with Medications
- Chapter 10: Everything You Need to Know about Nutrition and Type 2 Diabetes
- Chapter 11: Eating Out and Being Social
- Chapter 12: Exercise and Staying Active
- Section 4 (chapters 23–32): Resources for All

CHAPTER 1

SO, YOU HAVE GESTATIONAL DIABETES

"My first reaction was to cry. I was so scared for my baby and once I got over crying, I was mad at myself . . . I wish I would have known that even with gestational diabetes you can still deliver a perfectly healthy baby and have a beautiful pregnancy."

—Diana Diaz, diagnosed with gestational diabetes and mom of a healthy baby boy.

Gestational D-I-A-B-E-T-E-S. . . . Say WHAT?! You've just come back from your checkup with the doctor where, after drinking a super sweet drink, you were told you have gestational diabetes. Your heart is racing, and you are in panic mode. Of course, you immediately consult "Dr. Google" and find a million different articles from a million different sources, but thankfully, you come across this book.

Receiving a diagnosis of gestational diabetes comes along with a series of emotions: guilt, shame, fear, and plenty of misconceptions about the condition. Trust me, you are not alone. In fact, gestational diabetes is one of the most common complications during pregnancy. It is estimated that over 8 million women[1] have gestational diabetes, and the number continues to rise. Gestational diabetes rates are increasing parallel to the rates of obesity and type 2 diabetes. Around 5–10% of all pregnancies will be complicated by gestational diabetes. But there's also some good news: about 70–85% of the time,[2] gestational diabetes can be treated with lifestyle modifications, which include nutrition, exercise, and maintaining a healthy weight—all of which are covered in this book.

If you've recently been diagnosed with gestational diabetes, this section is for you. In this section, we will cover what gestational diabetes is and who is at risk. By the end of this section, you'll understand why it matters to keep your blood glucose in check, and you'll learn what foods to eat, how to check blood glucose, tips to help maintain a healthy weight, and all about the day of delivery. If you live with type 2 or type 1 diabetes and are pregnant or wanting to get pregnant, make sure to check out sections 2 and 3. And don't forget to read the last section, "Resources for All," which takes the theory into practice by debunking common myths and providing you with sample meal plans, ideas on best snacks, recipes, and more. But first, let's try to understand a little more about gestational diabetes.

What You Need to Know about the Screening Test for Gestational Diabetes (a.k.a. the glucose challenge test)

Glucose screening during pregnancy is usually done at the end of the second trimester, around weeks 24–28, but may be done earlier depending on your risk factors. The screening and diagnosis for gestational diabetes can be done in one or two steps. The type of test you receive will depend on your doctor and hospital practice, but both tests are acceptable as they look for the same thing: how your blood glucose reacts to a large dose of glucose.

Two-Step Test

First step (1 hour):
- There is no need to fast or prepare beforehand.
- You will drink a very sweet drink that contains 50 g of carbohydrate.
- You will wait about 1 hour and then get your blood drawn.
- Your doctor will provide you with the results in the next few days.
- If your blood glucose is too high, you will return for a 3-hour glucose tolerance test.

Second step (3 hours):
- You will need to fast for 8–12 hours before the test.
- Your blood will be drawn fasting, and then you will drink a very sweet drink.
- Your blood will be drawn every hour afterward for 3 hours.

One-Step Test

- You will need to fast for 8–12 hours before the test.
- Your blood will be drawn fasting, and then you will drink a very sweet drink that contains 75 g of carbohydrate.
- Your blood will be drawn at 1 hour and 2 hours afterward.
- Your doctor will provide you with the results in the next few days.

What Is It?

In short, gestational diabetes is "glucose intolerance," or high blood glucose, that only happens during pregnancy. Before pregnancy, you did not have diabetes, but during pregnancy, your body undergoes significant changes that affect the way your body produces insulin. The majority of diabetes cases during pregnancy are gestational (about 84%), and the rest are preexisting type 2 and type 1 diabetes. Unlike preexisting type 2 or type 1 diabetes, gestational diabetes goes away after delivery. Despite the differences in treatment among the three, all diabetes in pregnancies share a similarity in that they pose a challenge to moms.

About 70%–85% of the time, gestational diabetes can be treated with lifestyle modifications, which include nutrition, exercise, and maintaining a healthy weight![1]

A Quick Physiology Class

Diabetes affects your body's ability to process carbohydrates because of problems with a hormone called insulin. Insulin is a natural hormone in the body that allows glucose (sugar) to be processed and then moved through the bloodstream into your body's muscles, cells, and organs for energy. As a result, insulin keeps our blood glucose in range. Without insulin, this sugar would be "trapped" in the bloodstream, unable to be used as energy. Without insulin, we would not survive. (Yay for insulin!) In type 1 diabetes, the body stops producing insulin. In type 2 diabetes, the body still produces insulin, but doesn't use it properly and progressively loses the ability to produce it. This condition is commonly known as insulin resistance. Although your body is still producing insulin, your cells aren't responding to it in the way they should. If you think of insulin as a key that opens the door to your cells so that glucose can go in, insulin resistance tampers with the lock so that the key doesn't work as well as it used to.

During pregnancy, our bodies go through significant physiological changes. One of them is to produce hormones (estrogen, progesterone) to help our babies thrive. But the increase in these hormones interferes with insulin. Think of it like an unbalanced scale: insulin lowers blood glucose, hormones raise blood glucose. In fact, pregnancy is referred to as a ketogenic or insulin-resistant state. In this way, gestational diabetes resembles type 2 diabetes because pregnancy hormones cause insulin resistance, so your body has to produce more insulin to maintain normal blood glucose levels. During pregnancy, your body has to produce almost three times as much insulin or more. Gestational diabetes occurs when the body is not able to keep up with the increased demands for insulin. Does this mean that you will *always* have diabetes? NO! Remember, gestational diabetes occurs only during pregnancy; however, there is a higher risk for you to develop type 2 diabetes later in life (Table 1.1).

TABLE 1.1 Overview of Different Types of Diabetes

Type of diabetes	Pathophysiology	How it's treated
Gestational diabetes	Occurs only during pregnancy	70%–85% diet and lifestyle 15%–30% medications
Type 2 diabetes	Insulin resistance	Diet, lifestyle, exercise, medications (pills and/or insulin)
Type 1 diabetes	Autoimmune disease in which body stops producing insulin	Only insulin

Risk Factors

There are several risk factors associated with gestational diabetes. You may have some of them, or you may have none of them, but studies show that gestational diabetes is more likely to occur if any of the following apply to you:

- You are older in age (>30).
- You are overweight or have obesity (BMI >25 kg/m^2).
- You had gestational diabetes in a previous pregnancy.
- You are not physically active.
- You belong to a high-risk ethnicity such as African American, Latin American, Native American, Asian American, or Pacific Islander.
- You have a history of diabetes in the family (first-degree relative).
- You have polycystic ovary syndrome (PCOS).

How Is It Diagnosed?

The current recommendations are to screen all pregnant women for gestational diabetes at 24–28 weeks. A glucose tolerance test examines how well your body is processing carbohydrates. Remember that super sweet, kind-of-disgusting drink at the doctor's office? It's called glucola, and it contains a large amount of glucose. The sugar from the drink raises your blood glucose. If everything is working as it should, your body will release insulin, which will move the glucose from your blood into your cells. If your blood glucose does not go back down to a normal level after a couple hours, it's a sign that the insulin in your body is not working well enough. Gestational diabetes is diagnosed when any single blood glucose measurement meets or exceeds the following levels:

- Fasting: 92 mg/dL
- 1-hour value: 180 mg/dL
- 2-hour value: 153 mg/dL

You may be screened earlier for gestational diabetes (at the first prenatal visit) if you have any risk factors for type 2 diabetes, such as being overweight, a family history of diabetes, or PCOS. If you are screened and found to have diabetes in the first prenatal visit, then the diagnosis is type 2 diabetes and not gestational diabetes.

Why It Matters to Keep Your Numbers in Check

The ultimate question for all women going through diabetes in pregnancy is, *"Will my baby be okay?"* If you keep your blood glucose as close to normal as possible (target range), the answer is, "YES." Maintaining normal blood glucose during your pregnancy will be very important for both you and your baby. It might not always seem like a walk in the park to achieve this, but trust me, it's doable and so very worth it. Having good diabetes management matters, and here's why.

Risks for Your Baby
- Neonatal hypoglycemia (low blood glucose in infant)
- Fetal macrosomia (large baby)
- Shoulder dystocia (birth injury)
- NICU hospitalization
- Predisposition to be overweight or obese in later years

Risks for You
- Early or at-term cesarean delivery
- Preeclampsia
- Excessive weight gain
- Type 2 diabetes in the future

Risks for Your Baby

This part can be very scary to a lot of pregnant women, but we must discuss the potential risks associated with consistently high blood glucose. As they say, with knowledge comes power! Gestational diabetes affects your baby later in pregnancy, once your baby is already formed. As such, birth defects are not commonly seen in gestational diabetes. Women with pre-existing diabetes, however, may be at higher risk of birth defects because high blood glucose affects the baby during the formation process.

High blood glucose during pregnancy puts your baby at risk for excessive growth or having a large baby. Larger babies face their own health risks, including birth injuries, also known as shoulder dystocia and low blood sugar at birth, known as neonatal hypoglycemia. Your baby can develop low blood glucose right after delivery because it's been forced to produce extra insulin due to high blood glucose from you, the mom. Hypoglycemia at birth may require additional care in the intensive care unit. Think about it this way: consistently elevated blood glucose in pregnancy gives your baby too much energy (kind of like giving your baby too many sweets) and causes your baby to gain too much weight, creating difficulties at the time of delivery. High blood glucose during pregnancy can also predispose your child to be overweight and have type 2 diabetes in the future,[3,4] continuing the cycle of diabetes. Like my doctor said, having a "candy bar" (elevated blood glucose) once in a while is ok, but every day is problematic.

Risks for You

Understanding the facts and knowing how to manage diabetes during pregnancy can mean avoiding a C-section and delivering a healthy-weight baby. The rates of cesarean delivery among women with gestational diabetes are higher compared to those without diabetes.[1] High blood glucose during pregnancy increases the risk of preeclampsia, defined as elevated blood pressure and protein in the urine, which may prompt cesarean delivery. Another important risk for moms with gestational diabetes is the increased likelihood of developing gestational diabetes and type 2 diabetes in the future. The statistics show there is a 50% chance[5] of developing gestational diabetes in future pregnancies, and it's estimated there is up to a 70%[6] lifetime risk of developing type 2 diabetes. Keep in mind that excess weight is a risk factor for developing type 2 diabetes, and because gestational diabetes can cause more weight gain during pregnancy, it may be harder to lose the weight postpartum.

Key Takeaways from This Chapter

✓ Gestational diabetes is a type of diabetes that occurs in the middle of pregnancy and goes away after pregnancy.

✓ 70%–85% of the time, gestational diabetes can be treated with lifestyle modifications, including nutrition, exercise, and maintaining a healthy weight.

✓ The risk of high blood glucose can lead to larger babies, high blood pressure (preeclampsia), and a higher risk of C-sections.

✓ Having gestational diabetes creates a higher risk of developing gestational diabetes during future pregnancies and type 2 diabetes later in life.

✓ Exercising and maintaining a healthy weight can delay and prevent type 2 diabetes.

REFERENCES

[1] American Diabetes Association. *Standards of Medical Care in Diabetes—2020.* *Diabetes Care* 2020;43(Suppl. 1):S1–S212

[2] American College of Obstetricians and Gynecologists. ACOG practice bulletin no. 190: gestational diabetes mellitus. *Obstet Gynecol* 2018;131(2): e49–64

[3] Duarte-Gardea MO, Gonzales-Pacheco DM, Reader DM, et al. Academy of Nutrition and Dietetics gestational diabetes evidence-based nutrition practice guideline. *J Acad Nutr Diet.* 2018;118(9):1719–1742.

[4] Lynn P. Lowe, Boyd E. Metzger, Alan R. Dyer, Julia Lowe, David R. McCance, Terence R.J. Lappin, Elisabeth R. Trimble, Donald R. Coustan, David R. Hadden, Moshe Hod, Jeremy J.N. Oats, Bengt Persson, for the HAPO Study Cooperative Research Group. *Diabetes Care* Mar 2012;35(3)574-580

[5] Schwartz N, Nachum Z, Green MS. The prevalence of gestational diabetes mellitus recurrence—effect of ethnicity and parity: a metaanalysis. *Am J Obstet Gynecol* 2015;213(3):310–317

[6] Kim C, Newton KM, Knopp RH. Gestational diabetes and the incidence of type 2 diabetes: a systematic review. *Diabetes Care* 2002;25(10):1862–1868

CHAPTER 2

MANAGING BLOOD GLUCOSE

"I kept my blood sugars in check by changing my diet,
being active, and having a routine in place.
I really had to focus and work hard on my routine.
Once I had one, it made a big difference."

—Melissa Amengual Nava, diagnosed with gestational diabetes
in her second pregnancy and mom of two healthy kids.

While the risks of gestational diabetes may be scary, the good news is that they can be avoided by managing your blood glucose through nutrition, exercise, and/or medications. It will be challenging at times, but just like every other challenge in pregnancy, you'll get through it with the help of your healthcare team, your loved ones, and resources like this book! It's just temporary, and the reward of a happy, healthy baby will be worth it. In this section of the book, we will walk you through the steps involved in checking your blood glucose, including appropriate blood glucose targets, how to check, when to check, record keeping, and the different tools available to test your blood glucose. Last, we will highlight factors that could impact your blood glucose and provide scenarios that detail what to do in case they are high or low. So let's get started!

Blood Glucose Targets in Pregnancy

Based on the research, we know that the closer your numbers are to target range, the more likely you and your baby will be free from complications. Having tight control of your blood glucose will be vital in having a successful pregnancy. According to the American Diabetes Association *Standards of Medical Care in Diabetes—2020*, the goal is to have blood glucose levels under 120 mg/dL at the 2-hour mark after meals, and under 95 mg/dL when you wake up.

Target Blood Glucose Levels

- Fasting: <95 mg/dL and either
- 1-hour postprandial: <140 mg/dL or
- 2-hour postprandial: <120 mg/dL

There are several ways to monitor blood glucose. The first and most common is via finger checks with a blood glucose meter, which is done 4–9 times a day. Another way is via a newer technology called continuous glucose monitors (CGMs). CGMs are devices that allow people with diabetes to constantly monitor blood glucose without needing frequent finger checks. (Learn more about CGMs below and in chapter 17, "Diabetes Technology—Pumps, Sensors, and More."). You might not have heard of them if you are not taking medications since they are more commonly used by people with type 1 or preexisting diabetes who are taking medications. Yet using this wearable technology is shown to improve diabetes management.

Besides using a glucose meter, there is another common test used to evaluate blood glucose: the hemoglobin A_{1c} ($HbA_{1c,}$), commonly referred to as A1C. The A1C test measures the average blood glucose in the past 3 months and is expressed as a percentage. The higher the percentage, the higher the average blood glucose concentrations. It is an easy and practical tool frequently used for people to assess diabetes control and adjust as necessary. During pregnancy, however, A1C is not the most accurate indicator of glucose management as results will be skewed and can be lower due to the expanding blood volume during pregnancy. Still, as a reference, it's good to know your value. The aim during pregnancy is to have A1C as close to normal as possible, ideally under 6.5%.

A1C Ranges to Know

- Normal: <5.7%
- Preconception goal: <6.5%
- Considered diabetes: ≥6.5%

DID YOU KNOW? *Studies show that maintaining an A1C under 6.5% is associated with the lowest risk of congenital abnormalities in your baby.*

How to Check Blood Glucose

Checking blood glucose can be an intimidating task, but we've come a long way in this area. Fifty years ago, people with diabetes could only check glucose in the urine and only got a range, not a specific number. Thankfully, monitoring tools in diabetes technology have advanced, and you can now monitor your blood glucose in various ways. Finger-stick testing is the preferred way to monitor blood glucose; the easiest way is via a glucometer. There are alternate sites like the forearm and thigh; however, they may not be able to capture the rapid changes in blood glucose that occur during pregnancy.[1] And no, unfortunately, you can't check blood glucose by just breathing or detecting your sweat via a wrist band. We still rely on blood samples to accurately read the glucose in the blood.

Tips for Accurate Blood Glucose Checking

- Wash your hands with soap and water. Food residue can significantly affect the test!
- Make sure your hands are dry. Wet hands can dilute the blood and generate "false low readings."
- You can use alcohol pads, but they are not necessary as you will be doing this four to nine times a day.
- Avoid using hand sanitizers as they may impact blood readings and can also dry out your hands.
- Rub your hands before to ensure proper circulation.
- Avoid oversqueezing as this can affect blood glucose reading.
- Change the lancet after every use.
- Use the same glucose meter consistently.
- Keep the meter and test strips in a dry, cool area.

Glucose Meters (Glucometers)

The nurse, educator, or doctor might have shown you how to use a glucose meter to check your blood glucose. (If they haven't, ask them to!) Here are some key things to know and remember: Glucose meters measure blood glucose from a small blood drop. You can find many brands in any pharmacy, and they all involve the same process: a lancing device, test strip, and the monitor. To find the lowest co-pay, check to see which brand your insurance covers. Most glucose meters are covered by your insurance, but there are many brands, and ultimately your insurance will decide which one is covered. Keep in mind that every year or so, insurance companies might alternate brands.

Continuous Glucose Monitors (CGMs)

As mentioned previously, CGMs are the newest technology that has revolutionized the world of diabetes. CGMs monitor blood glucose in real time by sensing the glucose present in the tissue. Instead of individual finger sticks, a sensor is inserted just under the skin to measure blood glucose continuously. Sensors may be more suitable to detect both hyperglycemia and hypoglycemia compared to traditional glucose meters. There are several brands of sensors with slight differences. Some CGMs measure glucose levels continuously and give both a blood glucose value as well as a trend, meaning they will indicate if blood glucose is going up, down, or remaining constant. These devices can provide automated alarms or alerts to indicate a specific glucose level or changes in glucose values. Other sensors measure glucose continuously but only display the number when you scan the device with a reader or smartphone. This means you will not get alarms and will only get the glucose number when you scan it.

Knowing your glucose levels can significantly alter the course of treatment. Let's say the monitor indicates you are at 80 mg/dL and going down. This might prompt you to have a snack ready in case the reading continues getting lower. As I've said, knowledge is power.

You might not have heard of CGMs if you have gestational diabetes, and there is a reason for this. The jury is still out on the effectiveness of wearing a sensor in the pregnant population with diabetes, especially for those women not on any medication. The use of CGMs has been studied extensively in people with diabetes who are not pregnant, and it has been demonstrated that they've improved diabetes control without increasing hypoglycemia. For some high-risk women, like those with hypoglycemia unawareness, the use of a CGM can be a useful tool to improve A1C as well as reduce low blood glucose. Furthermore, the effective use of real-time CGMs in pregnant women with type 1 diabetes can improve A1C levels, time in range, and overall health outcomes in babies. Some trials in pregnant women with preexisting type 2 or type 1 diabetes have shown improved health outcomes like lower birth weight and improved glycemic control.[2,3] Make sure to talk with your healthcare team to determine if a CGM is the right choice for you. (See more in chapter 17, "Diabetes Technology—Pumps, Sensors, and More.")

When to Check

I always say, "The more you know, the better you are." Only knowledge will allow you to make informed decisions on how to best manage your diabetes. Pregnant women with diabetes will need to check blood glucose anywhere from four to nine times a day, which will include fasting blood glucose, 2 hours after a meal, and possibly before meals. But this will vary depending on your treatment. If you are on medications, you will probably be told to check blood glucose more frequently as the numbers are more likely to change. Blood glucose tends to peak about 60–90 minutes after the start of a meal, so it makes sense to test at the 1–2 hour mark after starting a meal to make sure blood glucose is in range. Postmeal values are more likely to predict having a large baby (fetal macrosomia); in other words, keeping your 2-hour blood glucose in range will have a more significant impact on avoiding excessive fetal weight gain than your fasting blood glucose. So, postmeal checks really matter for you! Checking blood glucose before a meal may be indicated for some women, especially if they are using insulin because the value will help dictate the amount of insulin given before a meal.

DID YOU KNOW? *Having normal blood glucose after meals will likely predict having a normal-weight baby. If you start seeing higher blood glucose after meals, make sure to contact your healthcare team.*

Record Keeping

Having lived with diabetes for 19 years, I can tell you that keeping logs of my blood glucose, medications, and food is my least-liked activity and by far the most time-consuming one. However, speaking as an educator (and not as a patient), keeping track of your blood glucose is the most surefire way to know if what you are doing is working. Usually you will be asked to write down your blood glucose by time of day, including notes on food eaten and any medications taken. (See an example log on page 91.) Diabetes is a 24-hour condition, so it requires a lot of self-monitoring. The more you know about yourself, the effects of certain foods, or even how a brisk walk changes your numbers will further empower you to make educated choices. Self-monitoring and record keeping will help you and your healthcare team determine the most effective way to manage and keep blood glucose in range, whether through diet, exercise, or medications.

Factors that Affect Blood Glucose Levels

It's easy to feel guilty when your blood glucose is above target. Most of us attribute it to something we ate that maybe we "shouldn't have." However, food (a.k.a. carbohydrates) is just one of around 22 factors that are known to affect your blood glucose levels (see Table 2.1 for more factors). Some of these factors, like the foods you eat, getting a good night's sleep, and exercising, are easier to control. Others, such as stress, hormones, or time of day, are harder to manage. It's easy to see food as the main culprit for our blood glucose, but here lies the complexity of diabetes management. It's not just about the foods you eat; it's about your environment, activity, and even biological factors like hormones, stress, lack of sleep and even time of day. In your record keeping, try to record as much detail as you can on things like stress levels, exercise, and sleep so you can get the whole picture.

TABLE 2.1 **Factors That Increase and/or Decrease Blood Glucose[3]**

Variable	Increase	Decrease
Biological	• Lack of sleep • Hormones • Stress • Illness • Menstruation	• Menstruation
Food	• Carbohydrates • Large amounts of fat/protein	
Activity	• High-intensity and moderate exercise	• Light exercise • High-intensity and moderate exercise
Medication	• Medication timing	• Medication dose • Medication timing

Source: Adapted from Brown, A. (2018). 42 Factors that Affect Blood Sugar. Retrieved May 2020 from https://diatribe.org/42factors.

Factors That Affect Blood Glucose
- Stress
- Carbohydrate intake
- Hormones
- Time of day
- Exercise
- Lack of sleep
- Medications

What to Do If Your Numbers Are High

If your blood glucose numbers are above target (≥140 mg/dL) after eating, first, there is no need to panic. I remember vividly how frantic I would be every time I had a high value because I felt I was putting my baby in danger. You can't look at diabetes during pregnancy as black and white. If you start obsessing over every single value that

TABLE 2.2 Reasons and Solutions for High Blood Glucose

Reasons	Solutions
● Too many carbs	● Check portion sizes ● Read labels
● Stress	● Walking ● Journaling ● Meditation app
● Need for medications	● Keep logs of food and blood glucose ● Talk to diabetes educator, nurse, or doctor

is not in target, you'll go crazy. Instead of focusing just on the value itself, try to understand the *reason* behind the number (Table 2.2). Treat every high value as a learning experience! Remember, it's not always related to something YOU did, but maybe the pregnancy process itself. Ideally, blood glucose 2 hours after meals should be under 120mg/dL. If readings are consistently around 140 mg/dL, we need to take a look at what you are eating, your exercise routine, and your medications, if any. If you are seeing higher blood glucose regularly for 2–3 days, make sure to speak to your healthcare team. Symptoms of high blood glucose include tiredness, hunger, blurry vision, and irritability, among others.

What to Do If Your Numbers Are Low

Hypoglycemia, or low blood glucose, is defined as blood glucose under 70 mg/dL, but keep in mind fasting blood glucose should be 95 mg/dL or under. In the case of gestational diabetes or type 2 diabetes not treated with insulin, you are less likely to experience low blood glucose. So low blood glucose is not so much of a worry as high blood glucose in women with gestational diabetes. However, if you are taking medications and frequently have blood glucose under 70 mg/dL, this needs to be addressed ASAP. Severe hypoglycemia poses a risk to you because it could cause you to fall or lose consciousness. Reasons for low blood glucose include too many medications, exercise, extended periods without eating, or eating minimal carbohydrates (Table 2.3). Symptoms of low blood glucose include tremors or shakiness, cold sweat, trouble concentrating, and irritability, among others.

Treatment of low blood glucose warrants the 15-15 rule for treating hypoglycemia: 15 g of fast-acting carbohydrate (Table 2.4), such as 1/2 cup of juice or 3–4 glucose tabs, and waiting 15 minutes before testing again. In the case of diabetes in pregnancy, you might not need the full 15 g of carbohydrate; 7–10 g may suffice to avoid overdoing it and going high afterward. Keep in mind that during a pregnancy NOT complicated by diabetes, the body will tend to produce lower blood glucose (a woman can be in the 50s and not realize it), especially in the morning. Managing diabetes during pregnancy is like walking on a tight rope—it involves a balancing act to keep blood glucose under 140 but above 70 mg/dL.

TABLE 2.3 Reasons and Solutions for Low Blood Glucose

Reasons	Solutions
• Too much insulin/medications	• Keep track of your blood glucose and medications • Talk to your doctor in order to decrease medications
• Very few carbohydrates	• Include slow carbs (carbohydrates high in fiber) in every meal and snacks (see more information in chapter 3, "What Can I Eat with Gestational Diabetes?")
• Nausea/vomiting early in pregnancy	• Sip on regular ginger ale and eat saltine crackers
• Too much activity/exercise	• Include a snack prior to exercising and even after activity

TABLE 2.4 Best Foods or Drinks to Treat Low Blood Glucose with 15 g of Carbs

Food	Carbohydrate (g)
3–4 glucose tabs	15
4–5 pieces of hard candy	15
4 oz juice	15
1 tablespoon honey	15

Ketone Testing

Ketones are the waste products produced when there is not enough insulin in the system. In gestational diabetes, ketones can appear if there is not enough carbohydrate or energy consumed. Your doctor might ask you to check for ketones in the urine if you are losing weight or your blood glucose levels are elevated. It is a simple urine test, usually performed in the morning, in which you will dip a ketone strip into a clear urine sample. The strip will change color after a few seconds. Afterward, you will compare the color of the strip to the container to determine if ketones are present. If ketones are present and your blood glucose is normal, this can be an indicator of nutritional ketosis. In other words, you aren't getting enough calories and carbohydrates in your eating plan. Nutritional ketosis is different than diabetic ketoacidosis (DKA), which is a very serious condition more commonly seen in people with type 1 diabetes or those that take insulin. For more information on DKA, check out chapter 25, "Managing Side Effects of Pregnancy—The Good, the Bad, and the Ugly."

Key Takeaways from This Chapter

✓ Expect to check blood glucose often (four to nine times/day), both before meals and 2 hours after meals.

✓ Blood glucose targets in pregnancy are <95 mg/dL fasting and < 120 mg/dL 2 hours after meals.

✓ Start keeping a record of what you ate, activity, and stress, and look for trends.

✓ Many factors will affect your blood glucose, including stress, hormones, lack of sleep, food, and activity.

✓ If you see higher values for more than 2–3 days, contact your healthcare team so they can troubleshoot and make the necessary adjustments.

REFERENCES

[1] American Diabetes Association. 14. Management of diabetes in pregnancy: *Standards of Medical Care in Diabetes—2019. Diabetes Care* 2019;42(Suppl. 1): S165–S172

[2] Draznin B (Ed.). *Diabetes Technology: Science and Practice*. Arlington, VA, American Diabetes Association, 2019

[3] Feig DS, Donovan LE, Corcoy R, et al. Continuous glucose monitoring in pregnant women with type 1 diabetes (CONCEPTT): a multicentre international randomised controlled trial [published correction appears in Lancet. 2017 Nov 25;390(10110):2346]. *Lancet*. 2017;390(10110):2347–2359

CHAPTER 3

WHAT CAN I EAT WITH GESTATIONAL DIABETES?

"Fruit was one of my cravings during pregnancy. Meeting with a registered dietitian helped me understand I could still have watermelon, but I needed to learn about portion sizes and timing of snacks."

—Diana Diaz, diagnosed with gestational diabetes and mom of a healthy baby boy.

B y now, you've probably googled "gestational diabetes diet" or "what foods can I eat with gestational diabetes." The reality is there is no such thing as a gestational diabetes diet. As a registered dietitian and person with diabetes, I understand that what you eat will be an integral part of managing your diabetes and ensuring a healthy and successful pregnancy. Nutrition is the cornerstone of gestational diabetes management. Yet diabetes is very much individualized—everybody's diabetes is different and responds differently to food. In talking with women with diabetes, I've learned that nutrition is the most confusing part of managing diabetes. Plus, the overwhelming amount of confusing information does not make it any easier. *Can you eat carbs? Should you go keto in pregnancy? Can you eat fruits if you have gestational diabetes?*

In this section, we will cover in depth what to eat when you have gestational diabetes. We'll discuss which foods affect blood glucose the most and review different approaches for eating a balanced plate. And if you still have questions afterward, make sure to check out the Q&A in the "Resources for All" section where we bust some common nutrition myths.

What this chapter will cover:
- Why you should see a registered dietitian
- What you can eat
- Which foods affect your blood glucose
- Planning meals and monitoring carbs—What should your plate look like?
- Distribution, portions, and timing of meals
- Best foods for pregnancy and diabetes

Why See A Registered Dietitian?

All pregnant women diagnosed with gestational diabetes should be referred to see a registered dietitian. Yes, I'm a little biased in saying this, but the research supports it! Individualized nutrition therapy will help you create a plan that works for you. The thing with diabetes is that "no two diabetes are the same." What works for one person might not work for another person, which is why keeping a close record of what you eat and your blood glucose will make it easier to understand the impact of that meal on *your* blood glucose.

Even though there are guidelines and best practices to help you get started, you need to find what works for you. Meeting with a registered dietitian will help you maintain an appropriate weight, keep blood glucose in check, and help you meet essential nutrient amounts for you and your growing baby. Plus, studies show that getting nutrition counseling by a registered dietitian early on can result in decreased hospital visits, insulin use, and perinatal complications, and increased likelihood of a healthy placenta and appropriate birth weight.[1] A registered dietitian can also help you build life-long healthy habits. Remember, gestational diabetes goes away after birth, but your risk for type 2 diabetes later in life (as well as your child's risk for type 2 diabetes), sticks around—all the more reason to change to life-long healthy eating habits. Use this time with a dietitian to learn healthy eating habits to prevent type 2 diabetes later in life. To locate a registered dietitian near you or to search by expertise, check out www.eatright.org/find-an-expert.

Goals of Nutrition Therapy

- Encourage a healthful eating plan to keep blood glucose in range.
- Achieve a healthy and appropriate weight.
- Promote baby's growth and well-being throughout the pregnancy.

Source: Adapted from Duarte-Gardea MO, Academy of Nutrition and Dietetics Diabetes Evidence-Based Nutrition Practice Guideline. 2018.

What Can I Eat?

"What can I eat?" is probably the number-one question going through your head right now (It's also the number-one question asked by all people diagnosed with diabetes). When it comes to nutrition research and diabetes during pregnancy, there is still a LOT that we don't know. Looking at the research, there is no one specific diet that has been studied or proven to work for *all* women with gestational diabetes; rather, there are *multiple dietary* approaches that can be helpful. Some of these include eating foods high in fiber, plenty of vegetables, and a Mediterranean-based eating plan to name a few. So, the good news is that you may be surprised to know the variety of foods you will be able to eat during pregnancy. Contrary to popular belief, diabetes management is not about carb restriction, but rather smart carb incorporation. Eating the right type, amounts, and distribution of carbohydrates will be critical in ensuring a growing baby and normal blood glucose. So, when I hear

about women eliminating entire food groups like carbohydrates, it makes me think of the important nutrition they could be missing.

Some basic do's and don'ts include the following.

Do's	Don't's (avoid)
• Incorporate more whole grains, high-fiber foods, lots of vegetables, healthy fats, and proteins	Avoid eating too many concentrated sweets, which provide limited nutrition
• Include plenty of nonstarchy vegetables as they will be low in carbohydrates and help you fill up	Limit processed foods that are high in fat or sugar
• Combine different foods. Follow the Diabetes Plate Method to help visualize a healthy meal.	Avoid eating large portions of just one food group as this will not help curb hunger or balance blood glucose
• Eat whole fruit, which provides plenty of vitamins, minerals, and fiber	Avoid liquid carbs (fruit juice) as they will be absorbed much faster than whole fruit. Yay to fruit, nay to juices!
• Adding fiber, protein, and fat to meals will slow down the peak in blood glucose	The more processed the food, the faster the peak in blood glucose

DID YOU KNOW? *Studies show that the more types foods you expose your baby to, the less likely he or she is to be a "picky eater." More reason to include a great variety of foods in your daily meal plans![3]*

What Foods Affect Your Blood Glucose

All About Carbs

In order to better answer the question of *"What can I eat?"*, it's important you understand *how* food affects blood glucose and *which* foods will affect your blood glucose the most. There are three main nutrients found in food: Carbohydrates, Proteins, and Fats. Your body needs all three of them in (a wholesome and balanced way) to function properly. You've probably heard of carbohydrates, but if you haven't, let's spend some time understanding this controversial nutrient. Carbohydrates will directly impact your blood glucose because they are broken down into glucose and give your body energy. Yes, carbs have a bad reputation in the world of diabetes, but you and your baby need this important nutrient.

A common mistake women make when they first learn they have gestational diabetes is to eliminate ALL foods that contain carbohydrate. Let's get one thing clear: *Carbohydrates are not your enemy!* You and your baby both need carbs as they serve as the body's preferred source of fuel. But you need to know *which ones* to eat, as well as *how many* and *when* to eat them. The amount, type, and distribution of carbohydrate are all significant in managing diabetes during pregnancy. The minimum amount of carbohydrate recommended for pregnant women is 175 g per day[4] to meet your baby's brain needs. Remember, carbs are the brain's primary fuel. This is why when people cut carbohydrates from their diet, they feel tired, irritable, and have a hard time concentrating.

Foods That Contain Carbohydrate

- Grains/cereals
- Fruit and juice
- Milk and yogurt
- Starchy veggies, such as corn and potatoes
- Sweets and snack foods (chips, cookies, desserts)
- Beans and legumes, such as lentils and chickpeas

Foods That Won't Have as Much Impact on your Blood Glucose

- Protein
- Moderate amounts of healthy fats
- Non-starchy Vegetables (see list below)

TIP: *Slow carbohydrates are those which include whole grain, high fiber which will be absorbed slower by the body*

Slow Carbs

Now that we understand carbohydrates, let's talk about which ones to include. When choosing carbohydrates, try to choose what I call "slow carbohydrates". This is not a scientific term, but one I like to use for carbohydrates that are high in fiber and nutrients. These types of carbs will fill you up, and provide the necessary vitamins and minerals, but will be slower to raise your blood glucose. Slow carbs include whole grains, fruits with plenty of fiber and legumes, such as lentils or beans which include protein and can help curb spikes in blood glucose. Eating foods high in fiber can slow down the absorption of glucose into the bloodstream because fiber is not fully broken down and digested. Foods with fiber take longer to raise your blood glucose; thus, preventing sharp spikes in blood glucose (more on fiber below). Carbs that contain protein like legumes, pulses and even sprouted bread can also be considered slow carbs because they will raise blood glucose much slower than highly processed foods made with white flour like pretzels, white rice, or others. But keep in mind that there are individual variations as well. The main point is to choose your carbs wisely, not deprive yourself of them.

TABLE 3.1 Slow Carbs vs. Fast Carbs

Meal	SLOW carb (CHOOSE THESE!)	FAST carb (AVOID THESE!)
Breakfast	• Oatmeal • Whole-grain bread • High-fiber cereal • Sourdough bread • 2% milk and yogurt • High-fiber/high-protein pancake • Whole fruit	• High-sugar cereal • Bagel • Pastries • Juice • Regular pancake
Lunch	• Quinoa • Whole-grain rice • Beans • Sweet potato • Peas • Edamame	• Fries • Sushi rice • Regular subs
Dinner	• Whole-grain pasta • Egg pasta • Sweet potato	• Instant rice • Instant noodles
Snacks	• Nuts • Fruits • Yogurt • Peanut butter • Pistachios	• Pretzels • Pastries • Dried fruit • Fruit concentrated in syrup

Fiber

Fiber is a type of carbohydrate that is found in carb-containing foods like fruits, vegetables, and whole grains. But fiber is unique in that it is not fully broken down and digested, so it doesn't raise blood glucose as other carbohydrates do. Because it is harder to digest, fiber can slow down digestion and absorption of glucose from other carbohydrates, preventing sharp spikes in blood glucose.

Fiber is an essential nutrient for pregnant women with diabetes for several reasons. First, fiber helps relieve constipation, which is a common side effect during pregnancy. Second, fiber keeps you fuller longer (yay!) and can play a role in curbing excessive weight gain. Last, and most important, for women with diabetes, eating foods high in fiber can slow down the absorption of glucose into the bloodstream, which means lower blood glucose after eating. So, when you hear claims like "avoid all white bread," this is the reason. When glucose is packaged with fiber, as it is in whole grains (as opposed to refined grains), it takes longer to digest and is absorbed into the bloodstream more slowly. Whole-wheat bread and whole grains remain intact and contain all the "roughage" in the grain. Pregnant women need about 28 g of dietary fiber a day. When reading a nutrition label, look for foods with at least 3 g dietary fiber per serving or more to help boost your intake.

DID YOU KNOW? *Fiber is best absorbed with water, so make sure you are drinking plenty of water to keep your digestive system going.*

Understanding Proteins & Fats

Proteins are the building blocks of life—the amino acids that make up our muscles, bones, cells, and support your amniotic fluid. (The amniotic fluid is the liquid inside your womb where your baby floats and lives.) Proteins have a minimal effect on blood glucose (unless consumed in very large amounts, and this is only seen in women with type 1 diabetes). During pregnancy, your protein needs go up, especially in the second and third trimester, to make up for your baby's growth. Protein is needed to support your expanding uterus and breast tissue, as well as the increase in your baby's blood supply. The daily recommended intake for pregnant women is 71 g of protein (or 1.1 g/kg of body weight). If you are having twins, protein needs go up even more: you need an additional 50 g of protein per day. Yet for most Americans, getting enough protein is not a huge problem since we generally consume more than enough in a day.[4]

Protein also helps to curb hunger and slow down the rise in blood glucose. Including a protein at every meal and even in snacks can help mitigate the peaks in blood glucose and keep you feeling full for longer. Protein is in both animal and plant-based sources (Table 3.2). Some plant-based proteins may also contain carbohydrates, so keep that in mind.

TABLE 3.2 Examples of Protein Sources

Animal	Non-animal/plant-based
Chicken	*Legumes
Turkey	Nuts
Beef	Tofu
Pork	*Beans
Eggs	*Quinoa
Fish/shellfish	
Milk/yogurt	

*Contains carbs as well

Fat

Fats will not generally raise blood glucose. In fact, fat plays a vital role in our bodies, and contrary to popular belief, not all fat is bad. The type of fat, as well as the amount, is important to keep in mind (Table 3.3).

TABLE 3.3 Examples of Fat Sources

Healthy fats (CHOOSE THESE!)	Not-so-healthy (saturated) fats (AVOID THESE!)
Nuts	Lard
Olive oil/canola oil	Bacon
Avocado/avocado oil	Trans fats (found in cookies, donuts, pastries)
Olives	Coconut oil*
Fatty fish (good source of DHA!)	
Chia seeds/flax seeds	

*A word on coconut oil: For all the hype, coconut oil may not prove to be a magic elixir. Foods high in saturated fat have been linked to heart disease. Coconut oil is predominantly a saturated fat (86% saturated, compared to 14% for olive oil), which is the main reason its use is controversial. Currently, the consensus among the nutrition community is that a tablespoon or so won't be harmful, but the scientific data do not support further claims. It's best to stick with olive oils, avocado oils, and other unsaturated fats.[5]

Healthy fats include plant-based oils, such as olive oil and canola oil. These contain monounsaturated, omega-3, omega-6, and polyunsaturated fats that play a vital role in supporting a healthy pregnancy. In particular, the omega-3 fatty acids docosahexaenoic acid (DHA) and eicosapentaenoic acid (EPA) have been found to support a healthy pregnancy and promote brain, eye, and cognitive health in babies.[6] Omega-3 fatty acids are also associated with a lower risk of preeclampsia and preterm labor.[6]

Because the body cannot make omega-3 and omega-6, we must consume them in food or via supplements. The typical Western diet lacks adequate DHA/omega-3, which is why most prenatal vitamins now include 300 mg DHA. Good sources of omega-3s include chia seeds, seaweed, walnuts, and sardines. Fatty fish, like salmon, is another excellent source of DHA; however, many women avoid fish altogether due to high mercury levels or food safety. Consuming two servings of low-mercury fish or 12 oz of fish per week is considered safe in pregnancy. The benefits of consuming fish during pregnancy outweigh the potentially harmful effects of mercury on the baby,[6] so make sure not to skip this excellent food. Just ensure it's a fish low in mercury. (See chapter 24, "Resources for All," for more information on DHA and low-mercury fish.)

But what about saturated fats? Saturated fats are found in animal products like lard, butter, cream, fatty cuts of meat, and cheeses, as well as tropical oils like coconut and palm oil. Saturated fat is strongly associated with increased risk of heart disease. Excess saturated fat may also increase insulin resistance and is linked to fetal overgrowth.[7,8] Keep in mind that foods high in fat are also high in calories, so consuming too many foods high in saturated fats can make it harder to maintain a healthy weight during pregnancy. This is why limiting this type of fat in your diet will be important to help you manage your weight and blood glucose.

What Should My Plate Look Like? Planning Meals and Monitoring Carbs

Because carbohydrate is the nutrient that will affect your blood glucose the most, you may choose to track the amount of carbs you eat. Generally, for women with preexisting diabetes or type 1 diabetes, counting carbs is a fundamental pillar of blood glucose management, since insulin is given based on the amount of carbohydrate consumed. For women with gestational diabetes, you may not *need* to count carbohydrates, but one thing is certain: understanding which foods contain carbs, in addition to portion sizes, will make it easier for you to plan your meals.

Your healthcare team might have given you a specific amount of carbohydrates to eat, but they might not have shown you how to count carbs. You can monitor carbohydrate amounts in various ways, from advanced techniques, like reading nutrition labels or using a scale, to simple techniques like using the Diabetes Plate Method or learning about carb choices. Let's discuss a few (see following page).

The Diabetes Plate Method

This is a simple and visually effective strategy to plan meals and manage your blood glucose by understanding how to portion your plate. The diabetes plate method changes the way we are used to plating our food—it emphasizes vegetables and reduces carbohydrate. Start with a 9-inch plate (about the width of a sheet of paper): half of it should be filled with non-starchy vegetables (see list on next page for examples), which are naturally low in carbohydrate and high in fiber and water. Divide the other half of the plate into two quarters. One quarter of the plate should include a lean protein like chicken, low-mercury fish, lean meat, or a plant-based protein; the remaining quarter of the plate will be a high-fiber, slow-carb food like sweet potatoes, whole-grain pasta, brown rice, or legumes. Simple, right? Ensuring half of the plate is filled with non-starchy vegetables will instantly cut out unnecessary carbohydrates, while the remainder is divided between a lean protein and carbohydrate-rich foods. What I love about this method is that you can practice it anywhere. If you are eating out in restaurants, at a friend's house, or at work, remembering this method will simplify your life.

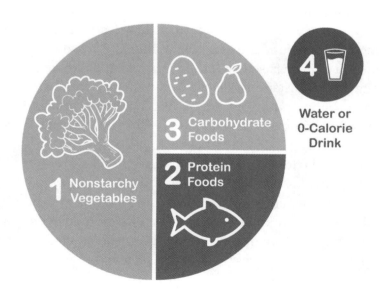

Key Points of the Diabetes Plate Method

- Fill 1/2 of your plate with nonstarchy vegetables.
- Fill 1/4 of your plate with carbohydrate-rich foods such as whole grains, fruits, starchy vegetables, low-fat yogurt/milk.
- Fill the remaining 1/4 with a lean protein.
- Include a small portion of healthy fat like avocado, olive oil, or nuts.
- Avoid sweetened beverages. Instead, drink water or non-caloric drinks.

Starchy Vegetables—Vegetables higher in carbohydrates. These are "carbohydrate foods" even though they are vegetables. Starchy vegetables include:

- Corn
- Potatoes
- Squash (Butternut, Winter, Acorn)
- Yam/Sweet Potatoes
- Peas
- Plantains

Non-Starchy Vegetables—Lower in carbs, usually higher in water content. They are a good source of fiber, vitamins, and minerals. The following is a list of common non-starchy vegetables:

- Amaranth or Chinese spinach
- Artichoke
- Artichoke hearts
- Asparagus
- Baby corn
- Bamboo shoots
- Beans (green, wax, Italian)
- Bean sprouts
- Beets

- Brussels sprouts
- Broccoli
- Cabbage (green, bok choy, Chinese)
- Carrots
- Cauliflower
- Celery
- Chayote
- Coleslaw (packaged, no dressing)
- Cucumber
- Daikon
- Eggplant
- Greens (collard, kale, mustard, turnip)
- Hearts of palm
- Jicama
- Kohlrabi
- Leeks
- Mushrooms
- Okra
- Onions
- Pea pods
- Peppers
- Radishes
- Rutabaga
- Salad greens (chicory, endive, escarole, lettuce, romaine, spinach, arugula, radicchio, watercress)
- Sprouts
- Squash (cushaw, summer, crookneck, spaghetti, zucchini)
- Sugar snap peas
- Swiss chard
- Tomato
- Turnips
- Water chestnuts
- Yard-long beans

PROS: The Diabetes Plate Method is the easiest way to create balanced meals with appropriate portions. There's no counting, measuring, weighing, or calculating needed.

CONS: With this method, you don't track the number of carbs or other nutrients. If your blood glucose levels are not in target, you might need to track your carb intake more carefully. Try one of the carb-counting methods below.

Reading Labels

Nutrition labels make it so much easier to count carbohydrates and monitor carb intake, so hooray for labels! The two most important things to understand are serving size and total carbohydrates.

First, look at the serving size. All the information in that label will pertain to the serving size highlighted. It can be 10 chips, 1/2 cup, or 3 oz. The manufacturers determine the serving size, so keep an eye on it as you may easily eat 2–3 servings if you are not careful. Second, look at the total grams of carbohydrate for that serving size. In my experience, people with diabetes start to get confused when they see the term "sugar" in the label and want to count it separately. But understand that the total carbohydrate amount accounts for sugar, starch, and fiber. For a more detailed explanation of nutrition labels and what to look for, check out chapter 26, "How to Read a Nutrition Label."

PROS: Reading labels is simple once you get the hang of it and can help you make informed food choices.

CONS: Not all foods have nutrition labels.

Serving Sizes/Choices

A nutrition label will show you how many carbohydrates are in that food or serving size, yet many foods like fruits, veggies, and certain grains don't always have a label. What do you do then? This is when learning about choices (or exchanges) will come in handy. The diabetes food choices are a list of seven different types of foods that are grouped and have similar amounts of carbohydrate, protein, and fat. One serving, or "choice," contains approximately 15 g carbohydrate. For example, one slice of bread equals 15 g carbohydrate, the same as one small apple. The idea is that you can then exchange one serving of carbohydrate for another of your choice while keeping the total amount of carbohydrate consistent. For more information on meal planning and carb counting, check out chapter 10, "Everything You Need to Know about Nutrition and Type 2 Diabetes."

Examples of One Serving/Choice (About 15 g) of Carbohydrate
- 1 slice of whole-wheat bread
- 1/2 cup beans or lentils
- 1 cup milk
- 1/2 cup cooked oatmeal
- 1 cup berries/strawberries
- 1/2 whole-wheat pita bread
- 15 grapes
- 1 small apple
- 1/2 banana
- 1 small peach
- 1/2 cup corn or peas

PROS: Choices can help you count carbs and other nutrients with more precision, but without having to carefully weigh and measure your food. You can also use it as a meal-planning method by determining your total carb choices per day and splitting them up in meals and snacks throughout the day.

CONS: You'll need special food lists or nutrition labels to determine the choices in different food items.

TABLE 3.4 Slow Carbs with Carb Amounts to Include in Your Diet

Slow carbohydrate	Amount of carbohydrate (g)	Carbohydrate servings/choices	Amount of fiber (g)
1/2 cup beans	15	1	7
1/3 cup oatmeal, dry oats (rolled oats/steel cut)	18	1	3
1 medium (5-oz) sweet potato	23	1 1/2	3–4
1/2 cup chickpeas (garbanzo), cooked	22	1 1/2	6
1/2 cup quinoa, cooked	20	1 1/2	2–3
1/2 cup lentils, cooked	20	1 1/2	7–8
1 1/4 cup whole strawberries	15	1	3–4
1 cup raspberries	15	1	8
3/4 cup blueberries	15	1	2–3
1 small apple	15–17	1	3
1 oz almonds	5	None	3–4
2 Tbsp nut butter (almond/peanut)	5–8	None	2–3

You can always use your hand and everyday household items to help you estimate portion sizes.

- Fist = 1 cup
- Palm of hand = 3 ounces
- Entire thumb = 1 tablespoon
- Tip of the thumb (to the first knuckle) = about 1 teaspoon

Using a Scale

A more advanced method of monitoring carbohydrates is to use a scale to determine the number of carbs per weight of a specific food. This method will be used mostly by women with type 1 diabetes or women with type 2 diabetes who are on insulin, as accurate carb counting will play a significant role in determining the correct dose of insulin to give.

PROS: You'll get a very accurate count of the carbs you eat at each meal, which can be helpful for dosing insulin.

CONS: Requires a lot of precise measuring and calculations, which can be a burden. If you're not taking insulin, this level of detail is not usually needed.

Using an App

When all else fails, you can always look up the nutrition content online or by using diabetes-specific apps. Note that the information online may not have been checked for accuracy and may be incorrect, so ensure you're referencing a trusted source. For a list of recommended apps, check out chapter 32, "Apps and Best Tools to Use."

PROS: Apps can make it much easier to more precisely track your carb intake as well as intake of other nutrients. Good for "guess-timating."

CONS: Nutrition information may not be 100% accurate. This method also requires tracking everything you eat in detail. While apps typically have extensive databases that include restaurant foods and packaged foods, it can be difficult to track homemade meals and foods.

Distribution, Portions, and Timing

"How many carbs can I eat?" "How often should I eat a snack?" These are common questions, and the answer is, "It depends." The amount of carbohydrates your body can tolerate is very individualized and is based on your weight, your body's reaction to insulin, and your medication regimen, among other factors. Excessive carb intake will make it more challenging to keep blood glucose in range; however, you also don't want to avoid all carbs since that can lead to ketosis. (See more ketone testing information in chapter 2, "Managing Blood Glucose.") Blood glucose checks should validate the number of carbs you eat and the distribution. In other words, your blood glucose checks will tell you if what you are eating is working.

Generally, a good recommendation is to limit carbohydrate intake to 35%–45% of your total calories from carbs, distributed among three meals and two to three snacks per day. So, if you are eating 2,000 calories a day, your approximate intake of carbs should be around 175–225 g/day. But remember that it's important to distribute those carbs throughout the day. The more carbs you have in one meal, the more it will raise your blood glucose. Furthermore, the time of day can also affect how your blood glucose responds to carbohydrates. For example, hormones that cause insulin resistance might be higher in the morning, leading to more elevated blood glucose with breakfast. Many women with diabetes will need to limit carbohydrates to 15–30 g at this time of day to minimize the peak after breakfast. In this book, you will find helpful meal plans ranging from 1,800–2,200 calories, depending on your needs. Carbohydrates will range from 30–60 g in each meal. Check out the sample meal plans in chapter 28, "Meal Plans and Tasty Recipes."

Sample Day

Breakfast: 1 whole-wheat English muffin with 2 oz cooked turkey breast, 1 slice mozzarella cheese, and 1/4 avocado + 8 oz almond milk + 1/4 cup blueberries (30 g carbohydrate or 2 carb choices)

Snack: 1 oz pistachios + 1 apple (15 g carbohydrate or 1 carb choice)

Lunch: 6 oz grilled chicken over mixed kale and spinach salad with 2/3 cup quinoa, 1/2 cup mixed fresh fruit (45 g carbohydrate or 3 carb choices)

Snack: 6 oz 1% vanilla Greek yogurt with 1/2 cup blueberries (18 g carbohydrate or 1 carb choice)

Dinner: 2/3 cup whole-grain pasta* with meat sauce and small side salad + 1/2 cup lower-sugar frozen yogurt (45 g carbohydrate or 3 carb choices)

(*You can make this dish with half zucchini-noodle pasta and half whole-grain pasta to add some veggies and increase volume without increasing your carbs!)

Snack: 1/2 pita bread with hummus, cucumbers, and tomatoes (15 g carbohydrate or 1 carb choice)

Keep in mind that food combinations and the timing of meals will also matter. Spacing your meals and snacks 2–3 hours apart can ensure you don't become too hungry and, at the same time, prevent your blood glucose from going too high or too low. Some women might benefit from three meals and 1–3 snacks a day. Keeping meals smaller throughout the day but adding snacks can also help prevent nausea or heartburn. Combining a carb with a protein or fat will slow down the digestion of glucose, so it's always a good idea to pair carbs with something high in fat and/or protein: a pita with hummus, an apple with peanut butter, or crackers with cheese (see chapter 27).

A Word on Glycemic Index

The Glycemic Index Diet was once popular in the diabetes community as a strategy to manage blood glucose; however, the reality is that it can be unreliable and impractical. The glycemic index (GI) measures how quickly foods that contain carbohydrates will raise your blood glucose. Foods are ranked from 0–100 and compared to pure glucose as a reference point (GI of 100). Foods with a high GI will release glucose rapidly into the bloodstream and tend to spike blood glucose. These include white rice, pretzels, baked potatoes, crackers, sugary drinks, pastries, and candy, among others. Foods with a low GI release glucose more slowly and can help keep blood glucose in a safe range. However, the GI refers to the *type* of carbohydrate but does not take into account the usual portion sizes, which we know are what really matter.

Additionally, GI can vary significantly if the food is eaten alone instead of with a fat or protein, and can also be affected by the cooking method. The literature concerning glycemic index and glycemic load in individuals with diabetes is complex, often yielding mixed results. In some studies, lowering the glycemic load of carbs demonstrated reductions in blood glucose. However, longer studies report no significant effect on blood glucose. So, the jury is not yet clear on using this approach. It can be useful to "fine-tune," but should not be used as the sole method to manage diabetes. A simpler approach is to focus on choosing slow carbs and reducing the overall intake of carbs.

Best Foods to Eat for Pregnancy and Diabetes

As you might have guessed by now, there is no "pregnancy diet" or "eating for two." However, during pregnancy, your body requires particular nutrients for your growing baby. What you eat during pregnancy will have a significant impact on the health and well-being of your baby. Consuming a wide variety of foods that include plenty of vegetables, slow carbs (like whole grains and fruits), and healthy fats will make it easier for your baby to receive essential nutrients like folic acid, calcium, fiber, vitamin D, omega-3, and DHA—all of which play a vital role in pregnancy. Do you need different vitamins compared to a woman who does not have gestational diabetes? No! The need for micronutrients like folate, vitamin C, and iron is the same as those for pregnant women without diabetes. The biggest and most crucial difference in gestational diabetes is ensuring your blood glucose is in the target range. That said, the portions of carbohydrates in each meal, the type of carbs, the timing and distribution of meals will be of great significance.

In terms of carbohydrates, 35%–45% of total calories from carbs could be a good start, but this can vary greatly. The best indicator will be your weight, blood glucose levels, and results from regular check-ups with your OB-GYN and diabetes team. A blood glucose test should validate whichever meal-planning tool you use. Let your finger checks be your guide. If you are under 120 mg/dL 2 hours after a meal and 90 mg/dL or less fasting, you are doing fantastic!

Below you will find some of my recommendations for top foods to include in your diet due to their unique nutrition profile for pregnancy. These "diabetes pregnancy superfoods" will ensure your eating patterns are balanced, nutrient-rich, and capable of preventing spikes in your blood glucose. There is an entire section dedicated to the essential nutrients you need during pregnancy in Section 4, "Resources for All." Here, you will find an in-depth discussion of special nutrients and supplementation like caffeine, folic acid, non-nutritive sweeteners. So, make sure you read it all.

TABLE 3.5 Best Foods to Include in Your Diet During Pregnancy

Food	Why it's so good
Salmon	Great source of essential omega-3, and high in vitamin D as well
Avocado	Healthy fat with omega-3 and lots of fiber, B vitamins, folate, and potassium
Sweet potatoes	High in fiber, vitamin A, and vitamin C, slow carb
Pistachios	High in nutrients, including fiber, fat, protein, potassium, and B vitamins
Eggs	Nutrient-packed, contains choline (25% of recommended daily intake), and high in zinc and protein as well
Berries	High in vitamin C and fiber, rich in antioxidants, and slow carb
Dark chocolate	Higher in fat and fiber and lower in sugar compared to milk chocolate, has polyphenols and flavonoids, which are antioxidants
Greek yogurt	A good source of calcium, vitamin D, protein, and probiotics
Apples	High in fiber, vitamin C, and slow carb
Nut butter	Healthy monounsaturated and polyunsaturated fats, high in fiber and protein
Dark leafy greens (spinach, kale, broccoli)	High in fiber, iron, calcium, folate, and potassium
Beans, lentils, legumes	Excellent source of plant-based protein, high in iron, folate, and calcium, slow carb
Sourdough or whole-wheat bread	Provides whole grains, and is a slow carb
Quinoa	Whole grain, rich in fiber, B vitamins, and high in protein, slow carb

Key Takeaways from This Chapter

✓ Carbohydrates will be important to monitor; knowing the type, amount, and timing will be the key to successful management.

✓ How much to eat is very much individualized based on weight, blood glucose, and activity.

✓ Focus on including a mix of slow carbohydrates, lean proteins, healthy fats, and fiber.

✓ Include plenty of nonstarchy veggies; fill half of your plate with them.

✓ Mornings might be harder to manage due to higher hormone levels; carbs may need to be limited depending on blood glucose after meals.

REFERENCES

[1] Shields L, Tsay GS, Eds. California Diabetes and Pregnancy Program sweet success guidelines for care [Internet], revised edition, c2015. Developed with California Department of Public Health; Maternal Child and Adolescent Health Division. Available from https://www.cdappsweetsuccess.org

[2] Duarte-Gardea MO, Gonzales-Pacheco DM, Reader DM, et al. Academy of Nutrition and Dietetics gestational diabetes evidence-based nutrition practice guideline. *J Acad Nutr Diet.* 2018;118(9):1719–1742

[3] Mennella JA, Jagnow CP, Beauchamp GK. Prenatal and postnatal flavor learning by human infants. *Pediatrics* 2001;107(6),E88

[4] Institute of Medicine. *Dietary Reference Intakes for Energy, Carbohydrate, Fiber, Fat, Fatty Acids, Cholesterol, Protein, and Amino Acids.* Washington, DC, The National Academies Press, 2005

[5] Neelakantan N, Seah JYH, van Dam RM. The effect of coconut oil consumption on cardiovascular risk factors: a systematic review and meta-analysis of clinical trials. *Circulation* 2020;141(10):803–814.

[6] Starling P, Charlton K, McMahon AT, Lucas C. Fish intake during pregnancy and foetal neurodevelopment—a systematic review of the evidence. *Nutrients* 2015;7(3):2001–2014

[7] Sivan E, Homko CJ, Whittaker PG, et al. Free fatty acids and insulin resistance during pregnancy. *J Clin Endocrinol Metab* 1998;83(7): 2338–2342

[8] Hernandez TL, van Pelt RE, Anderson MA, et al. Women with gestational diabetes mellitus randomized to a higher–complex carbohydrate/low-fat diet manifest lower adipose tissue insulin resistance, inflammation, glucose, and free fatty acids: a pilot study. *Diabetes Care* 2016;39(1):39–42

CHAPTER 4

MAINTAINING A HEALTHY WEIGHT AND STAYING ACTIVE DURING PREGNANCY

"Walking after meals helped me to bring my blood sugars down naturally."

—Emily Dudensing, registered dietitian diagnosed with gestational diabetes in all three of her pregnancies.

Weight gain in pregnancy can be a sensitive subject. *"Are you sure you're not carrying twins?"* (UGH!) I remember getting this type of comment in my second pregnancy, and I could just feel my blood start to boil. It's normal and expected for you to gain weight. After all, you are carrying a tiny human inside of you. The problem lies in gaining too much weight and developing gestational diabetes. Excess weight during pregnancy can lead to larger babies, as well as higher risk for a C-section and complications at birth. Although we don't know the exact cause of gestational diabetes, we know that gaining too much weight during pregnancy puts women at higher risk of developing gestational diabetes. That said, weight is only one risk factor; women who are not overweight can still get gestational diabetes. Other factors pertaining to genetics, maternal age, and specific ethnic groups remain, which is why all pregnant women are screened.

In this chapter we will talk about weight and pregnancy and what you need to know to stay healthy and active. We will review the latest exercise recommendations in pregnancy including best exercises and which ones to avoid. You'll learn helpful tips to stay on track with your weight and remain active. So, let's get moving! (Pun intended.)

Exercise Basics

"Can I exercise if I have gestational diabetes?" Yes! Exercise during pregnancy is widely accepted as safe, and is strongly encouraged in all women during pregnancy, especially those with diabetes. Being active during your pregnancy can help lower your blood glucose and reduces the chances of requiring insulin. Think of exercise like medicine—it makes the body more sensitive to insulin and helps the body burn carbohydrates (glucose) as fuel. Exercise is not only good for the body, but also the soul. It triggers the release of certain hormones that help decrease stress and is associated with an overall sense of well-being. Exercise can help prevent excess weight gain, reduce the risk of preeclampsia, decrease stress, and help keep blood glucose values in target.

Fortunately, exercise recommendations in pregnancy have evolved in the last 50 years, and they are not what your grandmother was once told. Previously, pregnancy was considered a disability, and women were told to avoid exercising as it was believed it could constrict blood flow and cause preterm labor. Now the opposite is true: the more active you are, the better for you and your baby. In fact, the American College of Obstetricians and Gynecologists (ACOG) changed its recommendations to state that women who were not exercising should start.

Not only is exercise recommended, but it's also used as a way to treat and prevent diabetes. The recommendation is to participate in

30 minutes of daily moderate physical activity, but this doesn't mean that you have to go to the gym for 30 minutes every day—it could be as simple as taking a brisk, 10-minute walk three times a day. Exercise should be individualized based on your current health and physical fitness.[1] If you do little or no physical activity, start slowly with 15 minutes of continuous exercise three times per week and gradually increase from 15 to 30 minutes. If you have never been active, now is not the time to start training for marathons. If you are on oral medications or insulin, you are at higher risk of experiencing low blood glucose. Timing of exercise, intensity, medication, and food intake before and after activity will need to be considered to reduce the risk of low blood glucose. (See more in chapter 12, "Exercising and Staying Active.")

Regular physical activity will reduce your risk of developing type 2 diabetes later in life, so take this time to make physical activity a daily habit and stick with it after delivery!

Benefits of Physical Activity on Diabetes in Pregnancy[1]

- Helps maintain a healthy weight
- Lowers blood glucose
- Reduces stress
- Increases and maintains strength
- Aids faster postpartum recovery
- Improves high blood pressure
- Relieves back pain

Best Exercises to Do in Pregnancy

The best exercises are those that do not pose a risk to you and your baby. Low-impact cardiovascular activities like yoga, walking, swimming, and riding a stationary bike are recommended during pregnancy. Contact sports like basketball, hockey, and football, as well as activities with a high risk of falling like hiking or skiing, are discouraged. Pregnant women engaged in upper-body cardiovascular activities showed lower blood glucose levels compared to pregnant women who solely followed a diet.[2,3] In fact, studies have shown that glucose metabolism is improved in only 4 weeks of engaging in constant physical activity, so a little can go a long way! If you are already active, way to go! You can probably continue your same routine with some modifications as pregnancy progresses.

Tips for Staying Active with Gestational Diabetes

- Try walking for 15–20 minutes after your largest meal (dinner).
- Avoid any contact sports that may pose risk for injury to you or your baby.
- Use the "walking and talking rule": if you can still talk while you walk, then your exertion level is appropriate.
- Try to include both cardiovascular and strength exercises.
- Take a walk during your lunch break. This will be a great way to help lower blood glucose after lunch.

Maintaining a Healthy Weight

Your pre-pregnancy weight, as well as how much weight you gain during pregnancy, will affect your baby's health. If you gain too much weight, you are at greater risk of requiring a C-section, increased water retention, and preeclampsia,[4] not to mention that it will be harder to lose that excess weight post-delivery. Furthermore, maintaining a healthy weight will reduce your risk of developing type 2 diabetes later in life. But remember that each woman gains at a different rate. Generally speaking, in the first trimester, we want to

TABLE 4.1 Target Ranges for Weight Gain

Pre-pregnancy BMI (kg/m²)	Total weight gain (lb)
Underweight (<18.5)	28–40
Normal (18.5–24.9)	25–35
Overweight (25–29.9)	15–25
Obese (>30)	11–20

Source: Rasmussen KM, Taktine AL (Eds). Weight Gain During Pregnancy: Reexamining the Guidelines. Institute of Medicine, National Research Council, Washington, DC. The National Academies Press, 2009.

keep the weight gain to a minimum (0–5 lb). As the pregnancy progresses, the weight gain should be gradual, with the last trimester showing the greatest gain. Your obstetric provider should closely monitor your weight gain. If you are gaining too little or too much weight, then a conversation should be started on what to do next (see Table 4.1).

What If I Am Overweight?

If you are overweight, pregnancy is not the time to focus on losing weight! Nevertheless, it will be beneficial to eat a healthy diet and slow down weight gain during pregnancy. Calorie intake recommendations can differ greatly depending on your pre-pregnancy weight along with your total weight gain during pregnancy. If you are at a healthy weight and follow an active lifestyle, you might be recommended to eat 2,500 calories/day; if you are overweight, you might benefit from lower calorie intake. Calorie and diet plan recommendations can vary significantly from woman to woman, which highlights why individualization and meeting with a registered dietitian are key. The results of some studies suggest positive outcomes in overweight women with gestational diabetes following a 1,500–1,800 calorie meal plan, but the evidence is not clear. There is no final calorie goal that women with gestational diabetes or even overweight/obese women should follow. Your focus should be on eating a healthy and varied meal plan that centers on wholesome foods with plenty of vegetables and whole grains.

To summarize, pregnancy is not the time to lose weight or be on a severe, strict diet. On the flipside, it's also not the time to "eat for two" and go on a calorie spree. How much you eat should be based on your activity, pre-pregnancy weight, BMI, and weight gain during pregnancy. Furthermore, your caloric needs will change throughout pregnancy. In the first trimester, your body doesn't really require additional calories or protein. You should continue with your current balanced eating plan. Starting with the second trimester, your calorie requirements will increase by an extra 300 calories/day, and your protein requirement will also increase to 71 g/day. The goal is to make sure weight gain is on track to avoid complications. Check out the meal plans in chapter 28, "Meal Plans and Tasty Recipes," to give you an idea of a typical day.

Tips for Maintaining a Healthy Weight

- **Eat plenty of nonstarchy veggies.** Veggies will help you feel full for longer because they are loaded with fiber and take longer to chew. Think about eating a bowl of broccoli instead of a bowl of cereal. If you're using the Diabetes Plate Method, make nonstarchy veggies half your plate.
- **Make snacks count.** Make sure you don't skip your snacks since they will help you curb hunger and maintain blood glucose throughout the day. Snacks should consist of slow carbs plus some protein and/or healthy fat to keep your blood glucose from spiking. (See chapter 27, "Best Snacks for Pregnancy.")
- **Take an after-dinner walk (15–20 minutes).** This is a great and simple strategy to stay active and help control blood glucose values after dinner.
- **Fiber is your friend**! Including foods high in fiber like whole grains, beans, and lots of fruits and veggies will equal cleaner, more wholesome nutrition.
- **Know your portions.** You don't need to eliminate rice or pasta; it's just a matter of knowing your portions. Try to use household measurements or your hands to remember the appropriate portions no matter where you are. This way, if you are in a restaurant, you'll still have a sense of your portion sizes and avoid overeating.

Key Takeaways from This Chapter

✓ Weight gain is expected. Everyone gains at a different rate, but keeping your weight gain steady will help you and your baby at the time of delivery.

✓ Now is not the time to start a diet, but it's also not the time to go on an eating spree.

✓ Make sure to double up on the veggies and make snacks count!

✓ Keep moving mama! Exercise is so beneficial for your blood glucose, not to mention it helps you avoid excess weight and keeps you sane!

✓ Aim for at least 30 minutes of activity daily.

REFERENCES

[1] Shields L, Tsay GS, Eds. California Diabetes and Pregnancy Program sweet success guidelines for care [Internet], revised edition, c2015. Developed with California Department of Public Health; Maternal Child and Adolescent Health Division. Available from https://www.cdappsweetsuccess.org/Guidelines-for-Care. Accessed 31 March 2018

[2] Jovanovic-Peterson L, Durak EP, Peterson CM. Randomized trial of diet versus diet plus cardiovascular conditioning on glucose levels in gestational diabetes. *Am J Obstet Gynecol* 1989;161(2):415–419

[3] Durak EP, Jovanovic-Peterson L, Peterson CM. Physical and glycemic responses of women with gestational diabetes to a moderately intense exercise program. *Diabetes Educ* 1990;16(4):309–312

[4] Werner E. *Medical Management of Pregnancy Complicated by Diabetes.* 6th ed. Arlington, VA, American Diabetes Association, 2019

CHAPTER 5

MEDICATIONS— WHEN DIET AND EXERCISE DON'T WORK

"Starting insulin does NOT mean you have failed.
It's not about you: it's the hormones."

—Reut Sher, nurse anesthetist and mom to two healthy boys.

You've been exercising every day, carefully keeping track of portions, reading labels, and eating wholesome snacks. And yet, your numbers are still too high. Yes, it happens. Even though in the majority of cases (70%–85% of the time) lifestyle changes alone can work to keep your blood glucose in check, you might fall into that roughly 30% of the population that needs a little extra help from medications. Remember, it's not always you: it's your hormones and the condition of being insulin resistant. In this chapter, we will discuss what to do when lifestyle and nutrition alone are not enough, and we'll cover the types of medication commonly used to lower blood glucose in pregnancy.

DID YOU KNOW? *There are about 22 known factors that can affect blood glucose. Pregnancy hormones are one of those factors that will be impossible to change. So, it's not you, or a failure on your end. It's your hormones!*

How Do I Know If I Need Medications?

Below are some factors to consider in determining your need for medications. As always, make sure to talk to your doctor before making any changes.

- You are seeing higher fasting blood glucose consecutively for 3+ days and/or have 6+ days of higher post-meal blood glucose.
- You are at higher risk due to having been diagnosed before the second half of pregnancy.
- You are at higher risk due to having been diagnosed with prediabetes before pregnancy.
- You have had a prior pregnancy with gestational diabetes.

Insulin

Insulin is the first-line agent for treating high blood glucose during pregnancy. For many, insulin has a bad reputation, and needing it is seen as a personal failure. As a person living with type 1 diabetes, I can tell you that insulin is what's keeping me alive. So, no, insulin is not evil! Would it be great to avoid injections? Of course! Nobody likes to poke themselves if they can prevent it. But in some cases, lifestyle changes might not be enough to control high blood glucose.

Insulin is the preferred medication for pregnant women as it does not cross the placenta, and therefore poses less risk for the baby. Furthermore, insulin has the longest track record because it's been studied the most in treating women with diabetes during pregnancy. There are several types of insulins available, including long-acting (glargine, detemir, degludec), short-acting (human regular), intermediate-acting analogs (human NPH), and rapid-acting (lispro, glulisine, aspart). Which one *you* use will need to be determined with your healthcare team as there is no guideline for a specific type of insulin to use. How much insulin you take will also be personalized and may depend on your weight, glucose values, and week of pregnancy. Understanding the types of insulin and how they work, along with individualizing medications, will be very important for you. Make sure to check out chapter 9, "Managing Blood Glucose with Medications," where you will find an in-depth look at the different types of insulin and how they work on your body.

Oral Medications

Unlike insulin, oral medications cross the placenta, and there is limited efficacy in using them as a *first* choice during pregnancy. Studies have been inconclusive in determining the long-term effects, which is why insulin tends to be the medication of choice. Keep in mind that the lack of long-term studies on these medications is because performing clinical trials in pregnant women can be very challenging due to safety and approval reasons.

The two medications frequently used in gestational diabetes when diet and lifestyle are ineffective are metformin and glyburide. These two drugs are often given as a first choice in people newly diagnosed with type 2 diabetes or prediabetes. However, during pregnancy, their recommendation may be more cautioned. Furthermore, even if you do take metformin or glyburide, there is a 20%–40% chance that your body will still require insulin due to higher-than-target blood glucose.[1] A 2008 study showed that about 45% of women treated with metformin during gestational diabetes ultimately needed insulin to achieve blood glucose targets.

There are cases, however, in which oral medications may be an alternative. Even though insulin is the most commonly used medication in diabetes and pregnancy, your OB-GYN may prescribe oral medications after determining exercise and nutrition have not worked. Oral medications provide some advantages: they can be less expensive and are easier to administer compared to insulin. Some women may not be able to use insulin effectively—whether it's due to cost, language barriers, or culture. But remember, no two cases of diabetes are alike. Make sure to have a conversation with your healthcare team to discuss the pros and cons of each medication so that you understand the risk and benefits. The following information will highlight some of the main points to consider when it comes to oral medications.

Metformin

- Crosses the placenta.
- A popular drug among people with prediabetes because it prevents the liver from producing too much sugar and improves the body's ability to uptake more glucose.
- Studies show that mothers who used metformin to treat gestational diabetes had children who were heavier in weight, had a larger waist circumference, and increase in fat mass 5–10 years later.
- Potential side effects include diarrhea, constipation, and cramping. Starting low and gradually increasing can usually resolve these gastrointestinal issues.
- Its use in gestational and type 2 diabetes is associated with less maternal weight gain, lower risk of neonatal hypoglycemia, and fewer rates of hypertension compared to insulin use.
- Almost half of the women on metformin may require insulin to achieve blood glucose targets.[2]
- Safe to use during lactation.

Glyburide

- Crosses the placenta and is associated with increased risk of infant hypoglycemia at birth (neonatal hypoglycemia).
- Long-term safety data for infants exposed to glyburide is not available.
- Improves blood glucose because it helps the body (pancreas) make more insulin.
- Side effects include hypoglycemia and increased weight gain.
- ACOG recommends it as a third-line agent following insulin and metformin.
- Safe to use during lactation.

TABLE 5.1 Overview of Metformin and Glyburide

	Metformin	Glyburide
What it does	• Lowers blood glucose by increasing body's use of glucose • Decreases excess sugar dumping	• Lowers blood glucose by increasing insulin production and sensitivity
Side effects	• Nausea, vomiting, diarrhea	• Low blood glucose • Weight gain
Possible benefits	• Associated with lower weight gain in pregnancy and less risk for hypoglycemia[2] • Less expensive than insulin	• Less expensive than insulin
Possible concerns	• Crosses placenta • Long-term effects in pregnancy with diabetes are unknown • Offspring had higher weight, BMI, and fat mass 5–10 years later	• Higher risk of hypoglycemia • Associated with larger babies • Crosses placenta • No known long-term effects

Key Takeaways from This Chapter

✓ Starting medication does not imply a failure on your end.

✓ Insulin is the preferred and most commonly used drug to lower blood glucose.

✓ Metformin and glyburide are the only two oral diabetes medications used in pregnancy.

✓ Long-term safety data of these oral medications (metformin and glyburide) are still unclear—in light of this, their use is cautioned.

REFERENCES

[1] Werner E. *Medical Management of Pregnancy Complicated by Diabetes*. 6th ed. Arlington, VA, American Diabetes Association, 2019

[2] American Diabetes Association. 14. Management of diabetes in pregnancy: *Standards of Medical Care in Diabetes—2019. Diabetes Care* 2019;42(Suppl. 1): S165–S172

CHAPTER 6

DELIVERY AND THE FUTURE AHEAD IN GESTATIONAL DIABETES

"It's not over just because you had a baby. Realize that you are at higher risk of gestational diabetes in future pregnancies, and type 2 diabetes later on in life."

—Alyce Thomas, registered dietitian, diabetes care specialist, and nutrition consultant at St. Joseph's University Medical Center, Department of Obstetrics and Gynecology.

Congratulations, you've made it this far! You have been looking forward to this day for a long time, and soon you will get to meet your baby. When I was pregnant with my first child, one of my main concerns was the actual birth. *Will I need to have a C-section? What type of monitoring will occur at the time of delivery? What will happen to my diabetes after my baby is born?* Having blood glucose numbers as close to target as possible will prevent you from unnecessary complications during delivery. In this chapter, we'll guide you through what to expect during delivery and after your baby is born. We will discuss blood glucose goals and the essential information to get you ready for the big day. Additionally, you'll find helpful tips on how to breastfeed successfully and balance life as a new mom. Delivering a healthy baby will bring the biggest joy and sigh of relief; all this hard work was worth it. Here you will also find important information to minimize the risk of gestational diabetes and type 2 diabetes later in life.

Blood Glucose Goals

During labor and delivery, the goal is to maintain blood glucose levels of 70–100 mg/dL. A paramount concern for women with diabetes during pregnancy, regardless of the type of diabetes, is the size of your baby. Large babies (also known as fetal macrosomia) can have trouble at delivery and cause shoulder dystocia, a birth injury that happens when one or both of a baby's shoulders get stuck inside the mother's pelvis. Furthermore, babies of mothers with diabetes are at higher risk of having low blood glucose (neonatal hypoglycemia) and may end up in the Neonatal Intensive Care Unit (NICU) to stabilize their blood glucose. Keeping your blood glucose in range throughout pregnancy and right up to delivery can help you avoid such complications and help your baby have normal blood glucose at birth.

Timing of Delivery

Thanks to modern advancements in diabetes monitoring, medications, and fetal monitoring, there is less need for early delivery. According to the American College of Gynecology, women with well-controlled diabetes can safely deliver vaginally, but this depends on several factors,[1,2,3] including the presence of complications and baby size (see Table 6.1). After week 32, your OB-GYN may want to keep a closer eye on you by looking for any signs of preterm labor, monitoring your blood pressure (risk of preeclampsia), and tracking the size of your baby. This might not be needed if your blood

TABLE 6.1 Delivery Timing Guidelines for Women with Gestational Diabetes

Diabetes control	Complications	Delivery
Well controlled by diet	None	39–40 weeks
Well controlled by meds	None	39 weeks
Suboptimal	None	37–39 weeks
Suboptimal	Significant	34–39 weeks

Source: Adapted from Werner, E. *Medical Management of Diabetes Complicated by Pregnancy, 6th Edition*. American Diabetes Association. 2019.

glucose remains in range and you show no signs of complication. Remember: the more in-target your numbers, the better for you and your baby.

If your baby is larger than expected, your doctor might want to induce labor or schedule a C-section ahead of time—usually around week 38—to avoid the risk of complication. But realize that what matters most is the health of you and your baby. I was not able to have a vaginal delivery, as I had hoped, due to my placenta previa, which is when a baby's placenta partially or totally covers the mother's cervix and therefore contraindicates a vaginal birth. And yes, I was very disappointed, but as my doctor told me, "Marina, welcome to parenthood—where you are not in control of everything."

Additional Post-Delivery Recommendations for Women with Gestational Diabetes[4]

- Women with gestational diabetes should have fasting blood glucose checked 24–72 hours after delivery to rule out hyperglycemia.
- Women with gestational diabetes should have a 75 g oral glucose tolerance test (OGTT) test 4–12 weeks after delivery to rule out prediabetes or diabetes. If normal, regular diagnostic tests should be repeated every 1–3 years.

Delivery: Testing and Monitoring

Your pregnancy experience will be very similar to that of a woman without diabetes. The main difference, however, is that you will be monitored more closely and may have more people in the room than you would like. Up until now, you have been regularly seeing your OB-GYN and are familiar with a nonstress test (where they place a fetal monitor on your abdomen and listen to your baby's heartbeat). During the delivery, your baby's heart rate will be monitored closely, and your blood glucose will be checked more frequently. If you are scheduled for a C-section, then you will get an epidural that will numb the lower part of your body. You will be surprised how fast the C-section operation will be. If you are on insulin, you will probably be placed on an insulin drip with dextrose (sugar) in case your blood glucose drops. (Check out chapter 21, "The Birth—It's Go Time!," for more information on what to expect during labor if you are using insulin.) Once you deliver your baby, there is a good chance your diabetes will go away, especially if you were well managed throughout your pregnancy. Nevertheless, your blood glucose will be checked soon after to make sure your numbers are in range.

Breastfeeding

All women should be encouraged to breastfeed because of the numerous health benefits known to both baby and mother, especially in the case of women with gestational diabetes (see Table 6.2). Research has shown that women who breastfeed are less likely to develop diabetes in the future.[5] Breastfeeding also helps you in various other ways: it helps you lose weight; it improves insulin resistance; it promotes a robust immune system for your baby; and it is associated with a lower risk of asthma, eczema, sudden infant death syndrome (SIDS),[6] diabetes, celiac disease, and other allergic conditions. Furthermore, breastfeeding is associated with a decrease

TABLE 6.2 Benefits of Breastfeeding

Benefits for your baby	Benefits for you
• Lowers the risk of allergic conditions (eczema, atopic dermatitis)	• Helps lose pre-pregnancy weight
• Promotes a healthy weight and lowers the risk of childhood obesity	• Improves insulin resistance
	• Returns uterus to regular size and reduces postpartum bleeding
• Lowers the risk of diabetes, celiac disease, and infections	• May lower the risk of breast and ovarian cancer
• Boosts baby's immune system and strengthens gut bacteria	• Saves money

in insulin resistance, which means improvement in the way your pancreas is working and a lower likelihood that you'll have diabetes in the future.

It's estimated that when you breastfeed, you burn an additional 400–500 calories a day, which is almost the equivalent of 1 hour of running. (Say WHAT?!) Meanwhile, breastfeeding also helps your baby by enhancing their immune system, promoting a healthy weight, and preventing future diabetes. But breastfeeding is not always as straightforward or as intuitive as it seems, and sometimes the added pressure to breastfeed can be very stressful. Successful breastfeeding will take practice, education, and determination. Don't be afraid to get help and seek the advice of a lactation consultant. If, for whatever reason, you aren't able to breastfeed, that's okay, too. A fed baby will always be a healthy and happy baby. And in the end, when moms are healthy, babies are healthy.

The Future Ahead

Be prepared: Once your baby is born, the hard work continues. Gestational diabetes may be over for now, but new challenges emerge: lack of sleep; a crying baby; changing diapers nonstop; and learning how to become a parent. Welcome to parenthood! We all know life is crazy with a newborn, but taking care of your health *now* is just as important as it was while you were pregnant. Your baby needs a healthy mom for the rest of her life! Remember, you now have a higher risk of developing type 2 diabetes, not to mention a 50% chance of developing gestational diabetes in your next pregnancy, so it's essential to maintain those healthy habits you worked so hard on during pregnancy! So, maybe it's not *really* over. The good news is you already learned everything you need to know to prevent diabetes in the future. Exercise and healthy nutrition will help make this possible.

It's important to check back in with your doctor 4–12 weeks postpartum to undergo another glucose tolerance test to make sure your blood glucose is back to normal and rule out a diagnosis of pre-diabetes or type 2 diabetes.[7] The glucose tolerance test (aka sweet-drink test) is more precise in detecting prediabetes and diabetes compared to the A1C test. The A1C is affected by red blood cells and overall blood volume, which is impacted during and after pregnancy and thus is not recommended to rule out diabetes postpartum. Keep in mind that gestational diabetes puts you at risk for developing type 2 diabetes later in life, so getting tested every 1–3 years and 4–12 weeks post-partum will be important. If your doctor has ruled out such diagnoses, there's no need to count carbs or diligently check your blood glucose anymore. All the same, maintaining the healthy diet and the exercise habits you started in order to manage gestational diabetes in pregnancy will still be beneficial to your health going forward. Losing the pregnancy weight can be one of the most helpful things you do to prevent both gestational and type 2 diabetes in the future. Gradual weight loss can be achieved through healthy eating and staying active. You can apply the same nutrition principles you learned here: slow carbs, vegetables, healthy fats, and lean meats. These are all part of a healthy diet that can reduce your risk of diabetes.

Balancing this new life is not easy, but it is important to take care of your health as well. Checking in with your doctor for an annual visit where they can test for type 2 diabetes will be beneficial. This can also be a good time to talk to your provider about contraception and family planning. Planning for pregnancy is critical in women who are at risk for gestational diabetes or developing type 2 diabetes. The biggest barrier for effective preconception planning is actually unplanned pregnancies. Because most pregnancies are unplanned, it's important for women with diabetes to have family options reviewed regularly to make sure effective contraception is implemented. This also applies to women in the immediate postpartum period. Just because you recently had a baby does not prevent you from getting pregnant. And no, breastfeeding does not act as a safe contraception method (in case you were wondering)! Women who have had gestational diabetes have the same contraception options and recommendations as those without a history of diabetes.

Tips to Help Prevent Gestational Diabetes in a Future Pregnancy

- Maintain a healthy lifestyle.
- Get to a healthy weight.
- Be physically active.
- Attend a yearly checkup with your provider to check fasting blood glucose as well as A1C.

Key Takeaways from This Chapter

✓ Your birth experience will be very similar to that of a woman without diabetes; the main difference is that you will be monitored more closely (blood glucose, baby's heart rate).

✓ You may not need to have a C-section. Women with well-controlled diabetes can safely deliver vaginally, but it will depend on other factors.

✓ After delivery, your blood glucose will return to normal and insulin resistance will go away, but you will need to follow up with your doctor 4–12 weeks later.

✓ Breastfeeding will help you return to pre-pregnancy weight and has SO many nutrition benefits for your baby!

✓ Because you had gestational diabetes, you are at higher risk for developing gestational diabetes in future pregnancies, and type 2 diabetes in the future. Use what you learned in this section to maintain a healthy and active lifestyle.

REFERENCES

[1] Spong CY, Mercer BM, D'Alton M, et al. Timing of indicated late-preterm and early-term birth. *Obstet Gynecol* 2011;118:323–333

[2] American College of Obstetricians and Gynecologists. ACOG practice bulletin no. 190: gestational diabetes mellitus. *Obstet Gynecol* 2018;131(2): e49–64

[3] American College of Obstetricians and Gynecologists. ACOG practice bulletin no. 201: pregestational diabetes mellitus. *Obstet Gynecol* 2018;132(6): e228–e248

[4] Blumer I, Hadar E, Hadden DR, et al. Diabetes and pregnancy: an endocrine society clinical practice guideline. J Clin Endocrinol Metab. 2013;98(11):4227-4249

[5] Stuebe AM, Rich-Edwards JW, Willett WC, et al. Duration of lactation and incidence of type 2 diabetes. *JAMA* 2005;294(20):2601–2610

[6] Hauck FR, Thomson JM, Tanabe KO, et al. Breastfeeding and reduced risk of sudden infant death syndrome: a meta-analysis. *Pediatrics* 2011;128(1): 103–110

[7] Werner E. *Medical Management of Pregnancy Complicated by Diabetes*. 6th ed. Arlington, VA, American Diabetes Association, 2019

Type 2 Diabetes and Pregnancy

SECTION 2
Type 2 Diabetes and Pregnancy

Helpful Chapters to Review

- Chapter 15: Preconception Planning and Goals
- Chapter 16: Strategies to Avoid Spikes in Blood Glucose
- Chapter 17: Diabetes-Technology—Pumps, Sensors, and More
- Chapter 18: The First Trimester—Congratulations, Baby on Board!
- Chapter 19: The Second Trimester—Bumpy Road Ahead
- Chapter 20: The Third Trimester—The Last Stretch!
- Section 4 (chapters 21–29): Resources for All

CHAPTER 7

THE BASICS

*"Don't freak out! You can do it; good glycemic control
yields good results. It's doable with knowledge, support,
and a commitment to maintain appropriate control."*

—Dr. Carlos Garcia, OB-GYN, Miami, FL.

I f you have type 2 diabetes and are thinking of having a baby (or have
a baby on the way) and don't know where to start, you've come to
the right place! In this section, we'll go step-by-step through what
you need to know to have a healthy and successful pregnancy. We'll
review blood glucose goals, pregnancy checklists, and exercise tips
in addition to helpful strategies to maintain tight blood glucose management throughout pregnancy. Last, we'll review medications used
to treat type 2 diabetes and learn what to eat and how to navigate the
restaurant scene. This section of the book is for the woman who has
already been diagnosed with type 2 diabetes before pregnancy—also
referred to as preexisting type 2 diabetes. You might also find very helpful information regarding what to expect in the first, second, and third
trimesters of pregnancy in the following section, "Type 1 Diabetes."

At the same time if you are on an insulin pump, you will find information that can apply to you in chapters 16 and 17. Finally, make sure to read the last section of the book, "Resources for All," where we include helpful information for *all* pregnant women dealing with diabetes. We will cover things like morning sickness, essential nutrients during pregnancy, managing stress, understanding nutrition labels, and debunking common myths in a Q&A chapter.

As if living with diabetes wasn't hard enough, pregnancy with diabetes adds a new dimension of complexity. You probably have a lot of doubts about how pregnancy will affect your diabetes (I know I did!). But I want you to know this: First, you can have a healthy baby. Second, it will take extra effort and dedication, but you can also have a successful pregnancy (and yes, it's worth it). Last, it helps to focus on what you can control. Many factors can affect your blood glucose during pregnancy, and they are not always in your control (e.g., pregnancy hormones). Diabetes management is not perfect, nor is it the same for everyone. Find what works for YOU! Get informed, be proactive, and remember to ENJOY this precious moment in your life. If you are feeling overwhelmed, check out chapter 29, "Managing Stress," and don't forget there are professionals that can help you. Don't let misinformation or lack of information take you into a state of panic. Make sure you read chapter 18, "The First Trimester"—*My Husband's Advice to Other Partners* (page 189), where he shares real-life advice from his perspective during our pregnancy journey.

Quick Review: What Is Type 2 Diabetes?

Type 2 diabetes is defined as "insulin resistance," which causes your blood glucose to be higher than normal. Some people can manage their diabetes with just healthy eating and exercise, while others need medication and/or insulin to help manage it. There is no right or wrong treatment, just as there is no one-size-fits-all diabetes care. The longer you have lived with type 2 diabetes, the more insulin resistant you are, simply because your body continuously works harder to produce appropriate amounts of insulin. Eventually, your pancreas gets "burned-out." More than 90%–95% of people with diabetes have type 2 diabetes, making it the most common type of diabetes. With more than 14.9 million women living with diabetes, the prevalence of diabetes in pregnancy is on the rise. Most of the increase is seen in gestational diabetes, but also in type 2 diabetes, due in part to the rising number of cases of obesity worldwide.

How Is Type 2 Diabetes Different from Gestational or Type 1 Diabetes in Pregnancy?

Both type 2 diabetes and type 1 diabetes occur independent of pregnancy and are usually diagnosed *before* pregnancy. For that reason, you'll often see the term "preexisting diabetes." Unlike gestational diabetes, which is only diagnosed *during* pregnancy and goes away once you deliver the baby, type 2 diabetes is a chronic condition that needs to be managed for life. In gestational diabetes, about 70%–85% of cases can be treated with exercise and nutrition,[1] which is not always the case for type 2; it's certainly not the case for type 1 diabetes, in which taking insulin is essential due to the fact that the body does not produce it.

Pregnancy is considered an insulin-resistant state. Women with preexisting diabetes may have a harder time managing diabetes because of the expected rise in insulin resistance caused by pregnancy hormones. Exercise and nutrition may no longer be enough to keep blood glucose in target or compensate for the body's increased need for more insulin. Preexisting diabetes will require constant diet and insulin adjustments. Regardless of the type of diabetes (gestational, type 2, type 1), the ultimate goal for all is to keep blood glucose as close to normal as possible. The risks of high blood glucose to the baby are similar in all types of diabetes.

How Does My Diabetes Affect My Baby?

When you live with diabetes, it's especially important to make sure your numbers are in check before pregnancy, as the first 3 months of gestation are critical in your baby's development. The goal is to keep blood glucose as close to normal as possible without enduring hypoglycemia. Consistently high blood glucose can put you and your baby at risk for serious health complications like preeclampsia, congenital abnormalities (heart defects), fetal macrosomia (large baby), neonatal hypoglycemia (low blood glucose at birth), birth trauma, or even spontaneous abortion.

One of the most critical periods for your baby is the first 14–56 days after conception. During this time, your baby's organs—the lungs, heart, brain, ears, and so forth—are being formed. The problem is many women don't realize they are pregnant until midway through their first trimester, meaning perinatal care will not begin until after week 10–12 when the critical formation period has passed. If you are overweight, have high blood pressure, or have any other chronic condition before pregnancy, it will be crucial to plan ahead and obtain the green light from your doctor to reduce any potential risks to your baby. And whether you have gestational, type 2, or type 1 diabetes, it's essential to keep your blood glucose targets in check before, during, and after pregnancy.

The good news is that planning for conception will undoubtedly have a positive impact on your health and reduce the likelihood of any adverse event. In the next chapter, we'll review in detail everything you need to know to get ready for pregnancy, including the preconception planning checklist, getting to know the pregnancy team, identifying and treating chronic complications, achieving a healthy weight, and more.

DID YOU KNOW? *By week 6 of pregnancy, your baby has already formed the neural tube, which is where your baby's brain is developing. By week 10, all major body organs are formed.*

Key Takeaways from This Chapter

✓ Type 2 diabetes in pregnancy is different from gestational diabetes in that it occurs before becoming pregnant and does not "go away" after pregnancy.

✓ The majority of diabetes cases are type 2 diabetes, which can be managed with a combination of lifestyle modifications, nutrition, and medications.

✓ The longer you have lived with type 2 diabetes, the more insulin resistant you are and the more likely you are to need insulin to keep your blood glucose in range during pregnancy.

✓ Consistently high blood glucose can put you and your baby at risk for serious health complications like high blood pressure, congenital abnormalities (heart defects), fetal macrosomia (large baby), neonatal hypoglycemia (low blood glucose at birth), birth trauma, or even spontaneous abortion.

REFERENCE

[1] American Diabetes Association. *Standards of Medical Care in Diabetes—2020. Diabetes Care* 2020;43(Suppl. 1):S1–S212

CHAPTER 8

GETTING READY FOR PREGNANCY

"My biggest advice for future moms with diabetes is to truly be ready to conceive. Don't rush into a pregnancy before you feel "in charge" of your diabetes control. If you know that you entered the pregnancy in a state of optimal blood glucose control, you will have less anxiety and worry less as you progress throughout pregnancy."

—Della Matheson, nurse and diabetes care specialist who lives with type 1 diabetes and is a mom to three healthy kids.

As with everything related to diabetes management, planning is vital, especially when it comes to having a baby. Preconception planning when you live with type 2 diabetes will ensure you have a healthy and successful pregnancy. Most important, being informed and empowered to make the best decisions for you and your baby will allow you to ENJOY the process. Ideally, preparing for pregnancy 4–6 months in advance is recommended to ensure your values are in check. Granted, life happens, and some pregnancies occur without a plan. In fact, about 50% of all pregnancies are unplanned, which makes it even more essential to know the risk and steps needed before becoming pregnant.[1,2]

In this chapter, we'll guide you through preconception planning (including blood glucose goals) and introduce you to the pregnancy team. We will also discuss ways to achieve a healthy weight and how to manage chronic complications before pregnancy. If you are already pregnant, congratulations! Follow along as we review blood glucose targets, glucose monitoring tools, and more.

What this chapter will cover:
- Pregnancy team
- Pre-pregnancy assessment
- Blood glucose targets and glucose monitoring
- Maintaining a healthy weight
- Managing preexisting complications

Getting to Know the Team

They say it takes a village to raise a child. The same can be said for managing diabetes in pregnancy. It takes a team approach to help you achieve tight blood glucose control and support you along these 9 months. Be prepared to have multiple appointments during this time, especially as you approach the last trimester. You might be visiting your OB-GYN and maternal-fetal medicine specialist or perinatologist twice a week starting at week 32, so make sure you get acquainted with them. You might not have access to all of these healthcare providers. Many places across the U.S. lack a multi-disciplinary team focused solely on diabetes and pregnancy. If you find a hospital that includes all the disciplines, you are in luck. But don't worry, you can always build your team and make it work for you. Let's first discuss who they are.

- **Endocrinologist**—A medical doctor specialized in treating diabetes and other endocrine disorders. If you are living with diabetes, you probably see an endocrinologist every

6–12 months. An endocrinologist is an integral team member as they are the diabetes "gurus" and will be monitoring your insulin regimen, labs, and diabetes control throughout your pregnancy. Make sure you pick one that is familiar with your needs.

- **Obstetrician** — Your OB-GYN is the "pregnancy doctor" who you will see very frequently. They will be the ones to actually deliver your baby and keep a close eye on ensuring that your baby is growing and thriving accordingly. When choosing an OB-GYN, you might want to ask what type of experience they have with women with diabetes. Ask about the labor and delivery process and how they usually manage women with diabetes in pregnancy. Make sure you feel comfortable asking questions and being honest with them, as you will see your OB-GYN every week near the end of your pregnancy.
- **Maternal-fetal medicine specialist (MFM)** — A high risk–pregnancy doctor, also known as a perinatologist. Many OB-GYNs don't work with high-risk pregnancy clients like women with diabetes, but instead refer them to an MFM. An MFM is highly specialized managing high-risk pregnancies, including those with gestational diabetes and preexisting diabetes. They will be doing more complex anatomy checks, assessing amniotic fluid, and performing fetal sonograms, among other complex exams. Depending on where you go, an MFM will see you weekly instead of your OB-GYN or endocrinologist.
- **Certified diabetes care and education specialist (CDCES or CDE)** — A certified diabetes care and education specialist is a person specialized in giving you the tools needed to thrive with diabetes. They will provide specific education to make managing diabetes easier. They can be a nurse educator, dietitian, nurse practitioner, or other trained professional. Make sure the CDCES you are seeing is experienced in working with pregnant women. In many offices, the nurse educator or CDCES will be the one closely following your blood glucose throughout pregnancy.

- **Registered dietitian (RD/RDN)** — The nutrition expert responsible for answering all your nutrition questions. It will be beneficial to meet with a dietitian before, during, and even after your pregnancy to review things like essential nutrients, the timing of meals and snacks, assistance with nausea, meal planning, carb counting, and more. If your doctor's office does not have one, you can find one by visiting www.eatright.org/find-an-expert.
- **Ophthalmologist** — A doctor who specializes in the study and treatment of the eye. Because pregnancy increases pressure to the eyes, you are at a higher risk of developing retinopathy. Make sure you visit the ophthalmologist to get a dilated eye exam before pregnancy, and then 3 months into your pregnancy to assess any changes.
- **Partner/significant other** — Yes, your partner will be a crucial player in this journey! It might seem obvious, but getting your partner involved early on in the pregnancy process is very important. If you're used to managing your diabetes on your own, your partner may not know the intricacies involved in diabetes care. Bring them along to the diabetes educator visit and teach them to check your blood glucose. It will be a good idea for them to know your signs and symptoms of low blood glucose. (See my partner's story in chapter 15, "Preconception Planning and Goals.")
- **Social worker** — A mental health professional who can help you navigate any financial, social, and psychological health needs. They can help you get the support you need, including locating a counselor or helping you navigate through your insurance so that you understand what is covered.
- **Lactation consultant** — A professional breastfeeding specialist who will help you breastfeed your baby successfully and support you if you experience difficulties. Some hospitals have lactation consultants on their services so you can ask to see one on your fist day after labor and delivery. You could also take breastfeeding classes beforehand to prepare you for what to expect.

Pre-Planning Appointment Checklist

- ❑ **Visit endocrinologist.** Discuss preconception blood glucose goals, review medications, get thyroid exam, screen for kidney disease, and obtain urine samples.
- ❑ **A1C under 6.5%.** The goal is to have A1C as close to normal and under 6.5% without the presence of low blood glucose.
- ❑ **Ophthalmologist exam with retina dilation.** Dilated eye examinations should occur ideally before pregnancy or in the first trimester, and then patients should be monitored every trimester and for 1 year postpartum, as indicated by the degree of retinopathy and as recommended.[3]
- ❑ **Dentist appointment.** The physiological changes during pregnancy put women at risk for dental problems such as cavities, gingivitis, and plaque. If you have diabetes, it will be important for you to visit your dentist for routine checkups.[4]
- ❑ **Keep and maintain blood pressure goals (<130/80 mmHg).** If you have high blood pressure, make sure to talk to your doctor about which medications are safe to use. (No ACE inhibitors.)
- ❑ **Take a prenatal vitamin with folic acid.** Begin taking at least 3 months before pregnancy.
- ❑ **Visit with CDCES and RD/RDN.** Discuss current medication and lifestyle treatment, evaluate patterns and trends, review important nutrients, discuss strategies for keeping blood glucose in target.

Pre-Pregnancy Planning

The goal of preconception planning is to normalize blood glucose before pregnancy and develop a plan with the necessary steps to get you ready for the big moment. Remember that the closer your blood glucose levels are to target before pregnancy, the more likely you are to have a healthy, successful pregnancy. During the preconception visit with your doctor or other healthcare team member, you will review blood glucose goals, A1C, medications to avoid, history and physical examination, and presence of retinopathy, renal, or cardiac issues. Particular attention should be given to insulin and oral medications, nutrition history, exercise, hypoglycemia unawareness, and diabetes monitoring.

Blood glucose targets are tighter in pregnancy compared to non-pregnancy. The goal is to keep blood glucose as close to 120 mg/dL as possible 2 hours after meals, with fasting values under 95mg/dL and an A1C under 6.5%. Achieving these targets might seem like an impossible task, but remember that the goal is not perfection. It is normal to have variation in your blood glucose, and you might not be able to achieve these values all the time. What matters is that you try to meet these goals as consistently as possible without significant hypoglycemia or hyperglycemia. If you need more tips to help you achieve these goals, make sure to read chapter 16, "Strategies to Avoid Spikes in Blood Glucose."

You should also meet with an RD to review your individual nutrition needs and ensure you are taking the appropriate vitamins and prenatal supplements. At this time, you should start keeping track of your blood glucose, foods, and medications to better understand trends and carbohydrate intake. You'll also want to review nutrition label reading and counting carbs, if needed.

Topics to Cover at Your Diabetes Prenatal Education Visit

- Pregnancy blood glucose goals.
- Monitoring goals for pregnancy
- What to do when blood glucose levels are high/low.
- Nutrition needs and carbohydrate monitoring/counting.
- Insulin management and/or medications. (Which are safe to take? Which to avoid?)
- Nutrient recommendations/important nutrients (folic acid, DHA, calcium, choline, and others).
- Checking for ketones. (When and where?)
- Food, insulin, and blood glucose logs.
- Meal plan review. (Food safety and evaluation of weight-gain recommendations and monitoring.)

Blood Glucose Targets and Monitoring

As per the 2020 edition of the American Diabetes Association's *Standards of Medical Care in Diabetes*, the fasting blood glucose goal during pregnancy is under 95 mg/dL, and the 2-hour postprandial (after-meal) goal is 120mg/dL. You probably already noticed that blood glucose targets are stricter during pregnancy compared to nonpregnancy. This is to prevent any complications caused by excess blood glucose affecting your baby. Before pregnancy, your doctor told you to aim for values under 140 mg/dL with an optimal A1C under 7%. But pregnancy is different. Your doctor will want you to have an A1C under 6.5% before getting pregnant. A target of under 6.5% is optimal during pregnancy if it can be achieved without significant hypoglycemia. The closer you are to these targets, the higher the chances of having a healthy and successful pregnancy. (See Table 8.1 for more target blood glucose levels.)

TABLE 8.1 **Blood Glucose Goals, Pregnancy vs. Nonpregnancy**

	Pregnancy	Nonpregnancy
Fasting	<95 mg/dL	80–130 mg/dL
1 hour after meals	<140 mg/dL	<180 mg/dL
2 hours after meals	<120 mg/dL	<180 mg/dL
A1C	Close to 6.5%	<7.0%

Source: Standards of Medical Care in Diabetes–2020. American Diabetes Association.

The first 8–10 weeks are critical for your baby's health because this is when the brain, lungs, spine, and organs develop (also known as organogenesis). Thus, the worry for women with diabetes is that if blood glucose is not well managed during this early period, there could be a potential risk of malformations. All the more reason why pre-planning is critical! Achieving values as close to target as possible is a realistic goal. But remember, just because you have a high blood glucose one day does not mean you are harming your baby. Blood glucose management is about the sum of its parts, not just one or two elevated blood glucose values. Keep that in mind throughout this journey.

What Is Hemoglobin A$_{1c}$?

The hemoglobin A$_{1c}$ (A1C) test is a blood test that tells us the average blood glucose level over the past 2–3 months. It is represented as a percentage. In pregnancy, A1C ideally should be under or as close to 6.5% as possible. Studies show that the closer you are to A1C <6.5% in the first trimester, the lower the risk of your baby having any congenital anomalies. [3,5,6,7,8,9]

When to Check Blood Glucose

You are probably already familiar with a glucose meter, but in case you are not, check chapter 2, "Managing Blood Glucose," for a refresher. It's recommended you check blood glucose in the morning (fasting) and after meals. In some cases, you might be told to check before and after meals, as in the case of women taking insulin who need to adjust medications. Expect to prick your finger about 4–10 times a day. The time of day you check is relevant as this will tell us how your body responds after certain foods and medications. Remember, the more you test, the more information you will have to make the best decisions. Checking at the 2-hour mark is ideal because food has enough time to be absorbed and reach its peak, and your results will give us a better idea of what is happening with your blood glucose.

When to check	BG goal
Fasting	<95mg/dL
1hr after meal	<140mg/dL
2 hours aftermeal	<120mg/dL

Keeping a Log

Unlike other chronic conditions, diabetes, for the most part, is managed by YOU. This is why self-monitoring is so important. The more you know about yourself, the effects of certain foods, or even how a brisk walk changes your numbers will empower you to make educated choices. Self-monitoring and record keeping will help you and your healthcare team determine the most effective way to control and keep blood glucose in range, whether through diet, exercise, or medications. Below is a sample log:

Sample Blood Glucose Entries and Notes

Week of March 4–8, 2019   = before meal   = after meal   = insulin/meds   = bedtime

DAY	BREAKFAST			LUNCH			DINNER			SNACK/OTHER	BED	
MON	83	173	5u	96	163	4u	174	143	8u	96	108	15u LONG-ACTING
TIME	8:45 AM	10:30 AM	8:45 AM	12:05 PM	1:45 PM	12:05 PM	6:15 PM	7:45 PM	6:15 PM	9:45 PM	10:15 PM	10:15 PM
Notes:	Big lunch — high-fat meal.											
TUES												

Continuous Glucose Monitors

Thanks to technology, we now have wearable devices that allow you to know your blood glucose level at all times without the need to repeatedly prick your finger. CGMs have revolutionized the world of diabetes because they measure glucose levels just under the skin, and with some sensors you can now see this data on your smartphone or device. The great thing about real-time CGMs is that they can provide you with alerts when your blood glucose values are high or low, and you can customize the alerts and targets. Some studies show CGMs may be more suitable to detect both hyperglycemia and hypoglycemia compared to traditional glucose meters. Additionally, some sensors allow you to share this information with other people, meaning they'll also be notified when your blood glucose goes too

TABLE 8.2 Pros and Cons of CGMs

Pros	Cons
• Data 24/7	• Higher cost
• Alerts for high and lows	• May not be covered by insurance
• Improved glycemic control	• May be overwhelming to have constant
• Less finger-stick checking	data on blood glucose
• Compatible with smartphone devices;	• May trigger fear of pain or discomfort
may allow you to share data with	• May result in adhesive reaction
other people	

high or too low. So, even when my husband was traveling overseas, he still received an alert if my blood glucose would go low. (See Table 8.2 for some pros and cons of CGMs.)

In general, CGMs consist of a sensor, transmitter, and receiver. CGMs monitor blood glucose in real time by sensing the glucose present in the tissue. The sensor is inserted just under the skin and transmits blood glucose readings every 3–5 minutes to either a small handheld receiver or your phone. Most can be worn for up to 10 days and provide about 288 measurements of blood glucose per day![10] When used *in addition* to blood glucose testing before and after meals, CGMs can help improve A1C targets in diabetes and pregnancy.[3] Continuous glucose monitoring metrics should not be used as a substitute for self-monitoring of blood glucose to achieve optimal pre- and post-prandial glycemic targets. However, wearing a CGM can decrease the frequency of glucose tests you perform, which is always a plus.

There are two different types of CGM devices: real-time CGMs and intermittently scanned CGMs. Real-time CGMs measure glucose levels continuously and give automated alarms and trends. Intermittently scanned CGMs measure glucose continuously but only display the value when you scan the device with a reader or smartphone; these kinds of CGMs will not give automated alarms. Furthermore, be aware that there are several brands of sensors with slight differences, as well. For instance, some CGMs give both a blood glucose value and a trend.

The best time to start with a sensor is before pregnancy so that you get familiarized with how it works. That way, you won't feel overwhelmed by the constant feed of information. If you're interested in learning more about sensors and technology, make sure to read chapter 17, "Diabetes Technology—Pumps, Sensors, and More."

Insulin Pumps

Although more often used by people with type 1 diabetes specifically, insulin pumps can significantly improve glucose management in people with preexisting diabetes. In pregnancy, they are safe to use and are associated with many benefits, including a decrease in hypoglycemia, better control of high blood glucose, and more flexibility. Compared to giving injections, a pump allows you to fine-tune basal insulin needs, facilitate corrections, and deliver insulin between meals or snacks.

However, insulin pumps are not for everyone, as they require a specific set of user characteristics. A person needs to be motivated and willing to understand advanced topics, as well as troubleshoot accordingly. Furthermore, the literature does not point out one mode of insulin delivery as being superior. The use of a pump versus giving injections in pregnancy has not been shown to yield significantly greater benefits. In a 2016 study[12] comparing insulin pumps versus injections in pregnant women with diabetes, they found only slight benefits in women wearing pumps versus multiple injections. However, it is worth noting that none of these studies evaluated the newest insulin pump models, which have come a long way since 2016 and have added features like stopping insulin if you are low.

So, the message is this: If you are wearing a pump, you can continue doing so; if you are on injections and can meet glucose targets consistently, then there is no need to change. However, if you are not able to achieve blood glucose goals and you feel like you can be a good candidate for wearing a pump, then it's worth considering.

Remember that the best time to start is well in advance, as there might be a learning curve. See more details about pumps in chapter 17, "Diabetes Technology—Pumps, Sensors, and More."

Achieving a Healthy Weight

Type 2 diabetes is often associated with excess weight. Since pregnancy is a state of expected weight gain, it's important to avoid gaining too much weight during pregnancy. Likewise, it's a good idea to consider losing weight *before* pregnancy to offset the potential risk. The recommended weight gain during pregnancy is the same for all women, with or without diabetes (and regardless of the diabetes type). Expect to gain about 0–5 lb in the first trimester and about half a lb to 1 lb per week after the second trimester. Again, each person is different. The weight gain recommendations are based on your weight before pregnancy (Table 8.3). In general, you want to gain weight very slowly in the first trimester. As you approach the second and third trimester, your baby will be growing rapidly. Expect to gain the majority of the weight in the last trimester.

TABLE 8.3 **Target Ranges for Weight Gain**[15]

Pre-pregnancy BMI (kg/m²)	Total weight gain (lb)
Underweight (<18.5)	28–40
Normal (18.5–24.9)	25–35
Overweight (25–29.9)	15–25
Obese (>30)	11–20

Being overweight raises the risk of high blood pressure, preeclampsia, and labor difficulties.[14] If you are overweight, it is ideal to lose weight before becoming pregnant. We know that even a moderate weight loss of 5%–10% of body weight can have a big impact on your diabetes management, as well as reduce your medications and improve heart health.[15] If you are already pregnant and overweight, the goal is not to lose weight or start a restrictive diet; instead, create a plan to promote appropriate weight gain. Working with a registered dietitian can help promote an individualized eating pattern, avoid rapid weight gain, and establish a physical activity routine.

Strategies to Help You Avoid Excess Weight/Slow Down Weight Gain
(see chapter 10 for more nutrition information)
- Increase intake of nonstarchy veggies
- Check portions
- Make snacks count
- Take a 15-minute walk after meals
- Include some resistance workout in your day
- Schedule nutrition consultation (weight-loss support groups, bariatric surgery)

How to Manage Preexisting Complications

Approximately 10% of all women (with and without diabetes) have high blood pressure, and the number-one killer in all women is heart disease.[2] Women with diabetes are at higher risk of developing chronic conditions like heart disease, high blood pressure, retinopathy, and kidney problems. The longer you have lived with diabetes and how well-controlled you are will play a role in developing complications. However, pregnancy can exacerbate diabetes-related complications, especially retinopathy and kidney problems. Certain medications commonly used to manage high blood pressure and cholesterol, including statins, ACE inhibitors, and beta-blockers, need to be discontinued before pregnancy due to the potential risk of birth defects. This is why it is crucial to get cleared before becoming pregnant, in addition to being closely monitored.

High Blood Pressure

The risk of hypertension or high blood pressure is higher in women with type 2 diabetes compared with type 1. In pregnant women with diabetes and high blood pressure, a target blood pressure goal of <135/85 mmHg is reasonable. Blood pressure should be measured at every routine visit, and targets may need to be individualized. During pregnancy, treatment with ACE inhibitors and angiotensin receptor blockers (ARBs) is contraindicated because of the potential birth defects they may cause in babies. High blood pressure drugs known to be safe and effective during pregnancy include: methyldopa, nifedipine, labetalol, diltiazem, clonidine, and prazosin. Always make sure to check with your doctor to see which medications will be safe to take during pregnancy.

Pregnancy after Bariatric Surgery

Many women may choose bariatric surgery as a way to improve their health. Compared to lifestyle efforts, bariatric surgery has a better response for treating type 2 diabetes. Pregnancy is also more likely to happen after bariatric surgery for women with type 2 diabetes.[16] The main issue to consider is waiting at least 12 months after having surgery due to the continual weight loss and nutrient depletion that occurs. Weight goals, carbohydrates, and calorie amounts should be individualized and based on your current weight. With careful monitoring, becoming pregnant after bariatric surgery can be safe and healthy.

Kidney Problems

Kidney disease is one of the leading complications of diabetes. If you happen to have any past medical history of kidney problems, pregnancy can worsen your kidney function. Because of this, all pregnant women with preexisting diabetes are checked for kidney health before pregnancy. Routine urine and blood labs are performed before conception and upon pregnancy to assess how well your kidneys are working. If you have a history of kidney problems, a nephrologist will closely monitor you.

Retinopathy

Pregnancy increases the risk of developing and/or worsening retinopathy. Retinopathy is a vascular complication common in individuals with diabetes that affects the nerves and lining of the retina, thereby affecting vision. All women with diabetes should be evaluated by an ophthalmologist to assess eye health prior to becoming pregnant. If no retinopathy is present, then you might be asked to return when pregnancy is confirmed to evaluate any changes that could have occurred during pregnancy. If retinopathy is present before pregnancy, then it might be best to wait until it can be treated and stabilized; otherwise, it might worsen during pregnancy. In the event you have retinopathy, you will be evaluated every trimester and 3 months after delivery.[17]

Key Takeaways from This Chapter

✓ Careful planning for pregnancy when you live with diabetes will be one of the most important steps to ensure a healthy and successful pregnancy.

✓ Diabetes can be complicated to manage, which is why having a multidisciplinary team to help you along the way will be key.

✓ If you are overweight and have type 2 diabetes, even a modest weight loss can benefit your pregnancy journey. If you are already pregnant, now is not the time to lose weight, but rather focus on a steady, healthy weight gain and include physical activity.

✓ Meeting with an RD and CDCES can help you lose weight and establish a healthy routine before pregnancy. During pregnancy, an RD/CDCES can provide you with an individualized meal plan with essential nutrients during pregnancy and can assist in nausea prevention, snack selection, and more.

✓ If you have a preexisting condition like high blood pressure, retinopathy, or kidney disease, it will be very important to get evaluated before pregnancy and get the green light as pregnancy can sometimes worsen such conditions.

REFERENCES

[1] Finer LB, Zolna MR. Shifts in intended and unintended pregnancies in the United States, 2001–2008. *Am J Public Health* 2014;104(Suppl. 1):S43–S48.

[2] Stang J. Preconceptions and Internal Nutrition Recommendations for Women with Diabetes. On the Cutting Edge, *Diabetes Care and Education.* 2016;Vol. 37(4):10–13

[3] American Diabetes Association. 14. management of diabetes in pregnancy: *standards of medical care in diabetes—2019. Diabetes Care* 2019;42(Suppl. 1): S165–S172

[4] Oral health during pregnancy and early childhood: evidence-based guidelines for health professionals [Internet], c2010. Sacramento, CA, CDA Foundation. Available from https://www.cdafoundation.org/Portals/0/pdfs/poh_guidelines.pdf

[5] Miller E, Hare JW, Cloherty JP, et al. Elevated maternal hemoglobin A1c in early pregnancy and major congenital anomalies in infants of diabetic mothers. *N Engl J Med* 1981;304(22):1331–1334

[6] Ylinen K, Aula P, Stenman UH, et al. Risk of minor and major fetal malformations in diabetics with high haemoglobin A1c values in early pregnancy. *BMJ* 1984;289(6441):345–346

[7] Greene MF, Hare JW, Cloherty JP, et al. First-trimester hemoglobin A1 and risk for major malformation and spontaneous abortion in diabetic pregnancy. *Teratology* 1989;39:225–231

[8] Eidem I, Stene LC, Henriksen T, et al. Congenital anomalies in newborns of women with type 1 diabetes: nationwide population-based study in Norway, 1999–2004. *Acta Obstet Gynecol Scand* 2010;89(11):1403–1411

[9] Bell R, Glinianaia SV, Tennant PW, et al. Peri-conception hyperglycaemia and nephropathy are associated with risk of congenital anomaly in women with pre-existing diabetes: a population-based cohort study. *Diabetologia* 2012;55(4):936–947

[10] Draznin B (Ed.). *Diabetes Technology: Science and Practice.* Arlington, VA, American Diabetes Association, 2019

[11] American Diabetes Association. *Standards of Medical Care in Diabetes—2020. Diabetes Care* 2020;43(Suppl. 1):S1–S212

[12] Farrar D, Tuffnell DJ, West J, West HM. Continuous subcutaneous insulin infusion versus multiple daily injections of insulin for pregnant women with diabetes. *Cochrane Database Syst Rev* 2016;(6):CD005542

[13] Rasmussen KM, Taktine AL, Eds. *Weight Gain During Pregnancy: Reexamining the Guidelines.* Institute of Medicine, National Research Council. Washington, DC, The National Academies Press, 2009

[14] Owens LA, O'Sullivan EP, Kirwan B, et al. ATLANTIC DIP: the impact of obesity on pregnancy outcome in glucose-tolerant-women. *Diabetes Care* 2010;33(3); 577–579

[15] Look AHEAD Research Group, Wing RR. Long-term effects of a lifestyle intervention on weight and cardiovascular risk factors in individuals with type 2 diabetes mellitus: four-year results of the Look AHEAD trial. *Arch Intern Med* 2010;170(17):1566–1575

[16] Chapmon, K. Bariatric Surgery, Pregnancy, and Diabetes. On the Cutting Edge. *Diabetes Care and Education.* 2016;Vol. 37(4):31–34

[17] Blumer I, Hadar E, Hadden DR, et al. Diabetes and pregnancy: an endocrine society clinical practice guideline. *J Clin Endocrinol Metab* 2013; 98(11);4227–4249

9

MANAGING BLOOD GLUCOSE WITH MEDICATIONS

"Insulin is not bad: it does not mean you have failed."

—Reut Sher, nurse anesthetist diagnosed with
gestational diabetes and mom to two healthy boys.

There are various ways of managing type 2 diabetes. One includes lifestyle changes; another is with the help of medication. Please note that lifestyle modification and medications are not mutually exclusive, nor is one better than the other. That said, some of the medicines you are taking to manage your diabetes may not be safe to use during pregnancy. In some cases, your doctor may want to start you on insulin. And no, insulin is not bad!

Insulin is the drug of choice for a pregnant woman with pre-existing diabetes (whether type 1 or type 2 diabetes), yet for some reason, insulin has a bad reputation. Of course, not having to inject is excellent, but starting insulin does NOT mean you have failed. Even if you are taking oral medications before pregnancy, there is a high chance you will require insulin to maintain normal blood glucose by the third trimester. During pregnancy, your placental hormones raise blood glucose, and your body requires almost triple the amount of insulin by the third trimester. Plus, the longer you have lived with type 2 diabetes, the greater the chance that your body (pancreas) is "exhausted," and might not be able to keep up with the increased demands of pregnancy.

In this chapter, we will review a list of common medications for managing type 2 diabetes in pregnancy (as well as those to avoid). We will discuss possible side effects and provide you with helpful tips to use medication safely. Make sure you speak with your health-care team about these medications so that you understand the pros and cons of each. For more information, check out chapter 5, "Medications—When Diet and Exercise Don't Work," and chapter 30 of the "Resources for All" section, "Q&A and Debunking Myths," where we touch on more on insulin myths.

When Will You Know If You Need Additional Medications?

As your pregnancy progresses, your insulin requirements will also change. In a healthy pregnancy, insulin requirements double by the second trimester and triple by the third. So, if you are already on oral medications to manage your diabetes, you might need insulin later on in your pregnancy to keep your blood glucose in target. If you follow a healthy meal plan and exercise, and are still unable to achieve blood glucose <120 mg/dL 2 hours after meals or <95 mg/dL fasting, you need to talk to your doctor about starting medications. According to the California Diabetes and Pregnancy Program, medication is required if you have three or more elevated fasting blood glucose values or six or more elevated after-meal blood glucose values in 1 week.[1]

If you are taking insulin before your pregnancy, expect to have multiple dose adjustments throughout your pregnancy. Finding the right amount of insulin is a real balancing act. Keeping a detailed record of what you eat, your medications, and your blood glucose will help you and your diabetes team fine-tune your doses as needed. Make sure to talk to your health provider before making any medication changes.

Insulin

Insulin is the first-line agent for managing diabetes during pregnancy. It is the preferred medication as it does not cross the placenta and poses less risk for the baby. It has the longest track record and has been studied the most in pregnancy and diabetes; many studies demonstrate its safety and efficacy. As a person living with type 1 diabetes, insulin has been a lifesaver. Literally! Without it, I would not survive.

Contrary to popular belief, insulin is not harmful to you or your baby. In fact, insulin is what allows your cells to use the energy in your body. Remember that during pregnancy, your body requires much more insulin, about three times as much in the last trimester. So, it might not be a surprise that you end up using insulin as your pregnancy advances. The goal of using insulin for the treatment of your diabetes is to help you maintain blood glucose in range without causing hypoglycemia. (This will require many adjustments to get the right balance.) There are several types of insulins available, and not all of them are approved for pregnancy. They are divided into rapid-acting, intermediate, or long-acting insulins (see Table 9.1).

DID YOU KNOW?

Before insulin was discovered in 1922, people who were diagnosed with type 1 diabetes did not live more than 1–2 years after diagnosis. Kids with type 1 diabetes would essentially starve to death because their bodies were unable to produce insulin and receive the energy their body needs. Now, thanks to insulin, people with diabetes can lead a long and healthy life free of complications!

TABLE 9.1 Types of Insulin

	What it does	Name	How it's taken	Onset of action	Duration
Rapid Acting/Mealtime/ Bolus Insulin	Provides fast coverage for meals/snacks and corrects high blood glucose	Lispro (Humalog)	Before meals and to correct blood glucose	15 min	3–5 h
		Aspart (NovoLog, Fiasp)	Before meals and to correct blood glucose	15 min	3–5 h
		Glulisine (Apidra)	Before meals and to correct blood glucose	15 min	3–5 h
Short Acting	Provides coverage for meals/snacks (no longer recommended)	Humulin R/ Novolin R	Before Meals	30–60 min	6–8h
Intermediate Acting	Provides intermediate background insulin	NPH	Twice a day	1–3 h	12 h
Long Acting / Basal Insulin	Provides background insulin	Detemir (Levemir)	Once or twice a day	1–2 h	12–24 h
		Glargine (Lantus, Basaglar, Toujeo)	Once a day	1–2 h	12–24 h
		Degludec (Tresiba)	Once a day	1–4 h	Up to 48 h

Source: Adapted from White, J (Ed.). 2019 *Guide to Medications for the Treatment of Diabetes Mellitus.* American Diabetes Association. 2019.

Mealtime/Bolus Insulin (Rapid-Acting Insulin)

Rapid-acting insulin, also referred to as bolus or mealtime insulin, is given to cover carbohydrates in the meal or to correct elevated blood glucose. It can be given by syringe, pen, or in an insulin pump. These types of insulin work fast (10–15 minutes after injection) and last about 3–5 hours in the system. The peak of rapid-acting insulins matches the time when blood glucose concentration peaks after meals, which is why this insulin is given to cover food. Additionally, it can be dosed more precisely and lasts for shorter periods. There are three types of rapid-acting insulins: lispro (Humalog), glulisine (Apidra), and aspart (NovoLog, Fiasp). Lispro and aspart are more commonly used in pregnancy. Another short-acting type of insulin, though not as fast as the previous ones, is regular insulin (Humulin R). Before rapid-acting insulins were available, short-acting insulin was given to cover meals; however, short-acting insulin is no longer recommended to be given at meals because it has a slower onset (peaks at 2–3 hours) and lasts longer in the system (6–8 hours). Rapid-acting insulins are the fastest insulins on the market. Compared to regular insulin (short-acting insulin), they are better at improving blood glucose after meals and reduce the risk of hypoglycemia.

Intermediate-Acting (NPH) Insulin

Neutral protamine hagedorn (NPH) insulin is also referred to as intermediate-acting insulin because it lasts in the body for 8–16 hours and starts peaking around 4–8 hours. It usually is given twice a day at breakfast and bedtime due to its peak times. It's less expensive than basal insulin, and some women may benefit from this regimen because it avoids an additional fast-acting (meal) injection. For years, NPH was the traditional insulin regimen used in pregnancy and type 2 until long-acting insulins become available and categorized as safe to use.

Basal/Long-Acting Insulin

Long-acting insulin, also referred to as basal insulin, provides slow insulin coverage that lasts in the body for up to 20–24 hours. It is given regardless of food, usually once or twice a day depending on dosages, and will not lower blood glucose rapidly. As with any long-acting or background insulin, the time of day you take it should be consistent to avoid any gaps in time. Both long-acting and intermediate-acting insulin can be used as basal insulin before and during pregnancy.

Detemir (Levemir) has been used more commonly in pregnancy; however, if you are using glargine (Lantus, Basaglar, Toujeo) before pregnancy, your doctor might keep you with this same medication. The newest long-acting medication is degludec (Tresiba). Degludec has a more extended coverage compared to glargine and detemir, with a duration of up to 30 hours. It's usually taken once a day and allows for more flexibility on the timing of the dose due to its duration. However, there are minimal studies that show the effects of this medication on pregnant women with diabetes. One study from 2018[2] suggested no identified risks in pregnancy, but there is limited data to show if its long duration may limit how quickly it can be titrated up or down. As always, make sure to talk to your doctor about the best type of background insulin for you.

Oral Medications

Before pregnancy, you were likely on some oral medication to help your body become more sensitive to insulin or help you produce more insulin. When diet and lifestyle modifications are not effective in nonpregnant individuals with type 2 diabetes, the next step is to start oral medications. Compared to insulin, oral medications are much more common in people with type 2 diabetes. However, during pregnancy, their recommendation will be more cautioned. Insulin is the preferred agent for the management of both type 1 and type 2 diabetes in pregnancy.

Oral medications cross the placenta (unlike insulin), and there is limited efficacy in using them as a *first* choice during pregnancy. Studies have been inconclusive in determining the long-term effects, which is why insulin tends to be the medication of choice. Keep in mind that the lack of long-term studies on these medications is because performing clinical trials in pregnant women can be very challenging due to safety and approval reasons. Other oral medications that will need to be avoided during pregnancy due to the risk of birth defects in the first trimester include high blood pressure medications, kidney-protective medications, and cholesterol-lowering and blood-thinning medications. Make sure to have a conversation with your healthcare team to discuss the pros and cons of each medication to understand the risk and benefits.

Medications to Avoid in Pregnancy

- High blood pressure medications (ACE inhibitors, ARBs)
- Cholesterol-lowering medications (statins)
- Blood-thinning medications (warfarin)

Key Takeaways from This Chapter

✓ Certain medications you might take to manage your diabetes and/ or other conditions like high blood pressure may not be safe to use during pregnancy.

✓ In a healthy pregnancy, insulin requirements double by the second trimester and triple by the third trimester.

✓ The longer you have lived with type 2 diabetes, or the earlier you were diagnosed with diabetes, the higher the chances your body might require insulin during your pregnancy.

✓ Insulin is the preferred and most common medication to lower blood glucose during pregnancy.

REFERENCES

[1] Shields L, Tsay GS, Eds. California Diabetes and Pregnancy Program sweet success guidelines for care [Internet], revised edition, c2015. Developed with California Department of Public Health; Maternal Child and Adolescent Health Division. Available from https://www.cdappsweetsuccess.org/ Guidelines-for-Care. Accessed 31 March 2018

[2] American Diabetes Association. 14. Management of diabetes in pregnancy: *Standards of Medical Care in Diabetes—2019. Diabetes Care* 2019;42(Suppl. 1): S165–S172

EVERYTHING YOU NEED TO KNOW ABOUT NUTRITION DURING PREGNANCY WITH TYPE 2 DIABETES

"You don't need to eliminate all carbs from your diet— you may be able to have rice, fruit, and milk. With the help of a registered dietitian, you can figure out how to reincorporate your favorite foods."

—Alyce Thomas, registered dietitian, diabetes care specialist, and nutrition consultant at St. Joseph's University Medical Center, Department of Obstetrics and Gynecology.

In today's diet culture, which is riddled with contradicting nutritional recommendations, it comes as no surprise that women with diabetes (and even pregnant women without diabetes) are so confused about what to eat. Pregnancy is a unique time in a woman's life when the body goes through a lot of physical changes. Proper nutrition plays an essential role in making sure both you and your baby are healthy. In these 9 months, your body will require certain nutrients to make sure your baby grows appropriately. But you might be wondering *"How will my diet will change once I become (or if you are already) pregnant with diabetes?"* *"Which foods are best to eat during pregnancy, and which should I avoid?"* *"Should I go low-carb in pregnancy?"* Rest assured, at the end of this section you will know the answers.

As a diabetes educator and registered dietitian, I can say with some certainty that food and nutrition are often the most confusing aspects of managing diabetes. You've probably already experienced this in your own diabetes management. As a person with diabetes myself, I understand that what you eat will be an integral part of managing your diabetes and ensuring a healthy and successful pregnancy. The goal is never restriction, but rather inclusion. To quote the Academy of Nutrition and Dietetics recommendation on pregnancy and nutrition "You should consume a wide variety of foods." Don't focus on what you *can't* eat; focus on what you *can*. It changes your perspective to a half-full glass mentality. I wholeheartedly believe pregnancy is a moment to be enjoyed as much as possible, including food that is delicious and wholesome, without compromising your diabetes management.

If you have found an eating pattern that works for you and has led to successful management, stick with it! There is likely not much that you will need to change during pregnancy. If you've been struggling to manage your blood glucose and feel you could be eating better, take this as an opportunity to explore new strategies and talk with a dietitian or diabetes educator if you haven't already.

In this chapter, we'll go from simple to advanced nutrition topics. First, we'll explore unique nutrient needs during pregnancy and highlight the best foods for you and your baby. We'll also do a quick review of nutrition and diabetes, particularly carbohydrates: where they are found and why it's important to monitor them, but also why carbs are essential for your baby's growth. You will also learn about "slow carbs"—what they are, and which foods fall into this category. Finally, we'll go in-depth into understanding portion sizes, timing, and the different ways you can monitor carbohydrates in your meals if that's something you choose to do.

What this chapter will cover:
- Nutrition during pregnancy
- All about carbs
- Portions, distribution, and timing

- Meal-planning and carb-counting methods
- Best foods for you and your baby

Nutrition During Pregnancy

What you eat during pregnancy will have a significant impact on the health and well-being of your baby. During pregnancy, your body will require particular nutrients for your growing baby. Some essential nutrients include folic acid, calcium, vitamin D, fiber, iron, and omega-3. There is an entire section dedicated to understanding these key nutrients as well as supplementation and food safety in "Resources for All," so make sure you don't skip it. However, you might be surprised to know that the same nutrition recommendations during pregnancy apply to you as to a pregnant woman without diabetes. In other words, the nutrients you and your baby need in pregnancy are the same as those for pregnant women without diabetes. The biggest and most important difference is that you will need to pay special attention to keep your blood glucose in range. The amount of carbohydrates in each meal, the timing, and the distribution of meals will be key in balancing your diabetes. Other key factors leading to a healthy pregnancy include:

1. Healthy pre-pregnancy weight
1. Appropriate weight gain during pregnancy
2. Eating a wide variety of foods
3. Supplementing with appropriate vitamins and minerals
   (See "Resources for All")
4. Safe food handling. (See "Resources for All")

All About Carbs

Either you love them, or you hate them. Yes, carbs have a bad reputation in the world of diabetes, but you and your baby need this important nutrient. Carbohydrates are the body's primary source of fuel and, as such, will have the most significant impact on your blood glucose. A common misconception during pregnancy in women with diabetes is that they need to eliminate ALL carbohydrates. Let's get one thing clear: *Carbohydrates are not your enemy*! You and your baby both need carbs as they serve as the body's preferred source of fuel. But consuming too many carbs might make it harder to keep your blood glucose in check. That said, you need to know *which ones* to eat, as well as *how many* and *when* to eat them. The amount, type, and distribution of carbohydrate are all significant in managing diabetes during pregnancy. As Goldilocks would say, "Not too hot, not too cold, just right!"

The Institute of Medicine recommends nonpregnant women consume 130 g carbohydrate a day, and this increases to 175 g per day during pregnancy to meet your baby's brain needs.[1] If you've ever tried to cut carbs, you might recall feeling tired and irritable or that you were having a hard time concentrating. That's because carbs are your brain's gasoline. Regardless of the regimen you follow or whether you are on insulin or not, you probably were told to balance your carbohydrate at each meal. In case you are looking to review basic but important concepts of nutrition and diabetes, check out Chapter 4, "What Can I Eat with Gestational Diabetes?"

Foods That Contain Carbohydrate

- Grains/cereals
- Fruit and juice
- Milk and yogurt
- Starchy veggies, such as corn and potatoes
- Sweets and snack foods (chips, cookies, desserts)
- Beans and legumes, such as lentils and chickpeas

Foods That Won't Affect Blood Glucose

- Protein
- Moderate amounts of healthy fats like olive oil, avocado oil, and nuts
- Nonstarchy vegetables (see list in the following section)

Slow Carbs

Now that we understand carbohydrates, let's talk about which ones to include. When choosing carbohydrates, try to choose what I call "slow carbohydrates." This is not a scientific term, but one I like to use for carbohydrates that are high in fiber and nutrient dense. These include whole grains, fruits with plenty of fiber, and legumes, such as lentils or beans, which include protein and can help curb spikes in blood glucose.

Eating foods high in fiber can slow down the absorption of glucose into the bloodstream because fiber is not fully broken down and digested. Foods with fiber take longer to raise your blood glucose; thus, preventing sharp spikes in blood glucose. (Not to mention fiber will help with constipation, which is a common side effect during pregnancy). So, when you hear claims like "avoid all white bread," this is the reason: White bread lacks fiber. When glucose is packaged with fiber, as it is in whole grains (as opposed to refined grains), it takes longer to digest and is absorbed into the bloodstream more slowly. Furthermore, carbs like legumes, pulses (edible seeds of plants in the legume family), and even sprouted bread also contain protein, which raises blood glucose much slower than highly processed foods like pretzels, white rice, or others. But keep in mind that there are individual variations, as well. The main point is to choose your carbs wisely, not deprive yourself of them.

TABLE 10.1 **Slow Carbs with Carb Amounts and Fiber to Include in Your Diet**

Slow carbohydrate	Amount of carbohydrate (g)	Carbohydrate servings/choices	Amount of fiber (g)
1/2 cup beans	15	1	7
1/3 cup oatmeal, dry oats (rolled oats/steel cut)	18	1	3
1 medium (5-oz) sweet potato	23	1 1/2	3–4
1/2 cup chickpeas (garbanzo beans), cooked	22	1 1/2	6
1/2 cup quinoa, cooked	20	1 1/2	2–3
1/2 cup lentils, cooked	20	1 1/2	7–8
1 1/4 whole strawberries	15	1	3–4
1 cup raspberries	15	1	8
3/4 cup blueberries	15	1	2–3
1 small apple	15–17	1	3
1 oz almonds	5	None	3–4
2 Tbsp nut butter (almond/peanut)	5–8	None	2–3

A Word on the Glycemic Index

The glycemic index diet was once popular in the diabetes community as a strategy to manage blood glucose; however, the reality is that it can be unreliable and impractical. The glycemic index (GI) measures how quickly foods that contain carbohydrates will raise your blood glucose. Foods are ranked from 0–100 and compared to pure glucose as a reference point (GI of 100). Foods with a high GI will release glucose rapidly and tend to spike blood glucose. These include white rice, pretzels, baked potatoes, crackers, sugary drinks, pastries, and candy, among others. Foods with a low GI release glucose more slowly and can help keep blood glucose in a safe range. However, the GI refers to the *type* of carbohydrate but does not take into account the usual *portion sizes*—which we know can really make a difference.

Additionally, glycemic index can vary if carbs are eaten alone versus combined with a fat or protein and can also be affected by the cooking method. The literature concerning glycemic index and glycemic load in individuals with diabetes is complex, often yielding mixed results. In some studies, lowering the glycemic load of carbs demonstrated reductions in blood glucose. However, longer studies report no significant effect on blood glucose. So, the jury is not yet clear on using this approach. It can be useful to "fine-tune" blood glucose but should not be used as the sole method to manage diabetes. A simpler approach is to focus on choosing slow carbs and reducing the overall intake of carbs.

What About the Keto Diet?

The popular ketogenic diet is based on eliminating all carbohydrates and eating a very high-fat diet with moderate protein (75% calories coming from fat, 20% from protein, and only 5% from carbs). According to research and healthcare experts, going keto during pregnancy is not safe or recommended. The ultimate goal of this trendy diet is to be in a state of nutritional ketosis. Ketones can be very dangerous in individuals with diabetes. Some studies done in pregnant mice following a keto diet have shown their babies had growth problems and even organ dysfunction. Now is NOT the time to go keto! However, if you were following a keto or very low–carb diet before pregnancy, you might want to meet with a registered dietitian, diabetes educator, or talk to your doctor to understand how to include carbs safely back into your eating plan. Keep in mind that reducing overall carbohydrate intake for individuals with diabetes has demonstrated evidence for improving glycemia and may be applied to a variety of eating patterns. Still, the message is that it's not necessary to avoid all carbs. The amount, type, and distribution will matter, which brings us to the next point: meal planning, portions, timing, and counting carbs.

Portions and Timing

How many carbs can I eat?

"How many carbs can I eat?" "How often should I eat a snack?" These are common questions, and the answer is, "It depends." The amount of carbohydrates your body can tolerate is very much individualized and based on your weight, your body's reaction to insulin, and your medication regimen, among other factors. You will probably need to be very mindful of carbohydrate intake, as this affects your blood glucose the most. Depending on what your carb intake was before your pregnancy, you may need to increase or decrease your carb intake. In women with diabetes, carbohydrate amounts are usually limited to 40%–60% of total calories. In pregnancy, a good recommendation is to aim for 35%–45% of your calories from carbs, distributed among three meals and two to three snacks per day. So, if you are eating 2,000 calories a day, your approximate intake of carbs should be around 175–225 g/day. Your needs will depend on your activity level and your current weight, among other factors.

Additionally, your carb needs may change throughout your pregnancy. Keep in mind these are general guidelines that can help you get started. Meeting with a registered dietitian nutritionist can be the best way to know the correct amounts to eat. In this book, you will find helpful meal plans ranging from 1,800–2,200 calories, depending on your needs. Carbohydrates will range from 30–60 g in each meal. Check out sample meal plans in chapter 28, "Meal Plans and Tasty Recipes."

If you were already used to following a low-carb eating plan before pregnancy, then you might be okay following the lower end of carbohydrate recommendation (again, not *eliminating* carbs). Your healthcare team will be following up on your blood glucose goals and weight gain to ensure your baby is growing appropriately. In case you are not gaining enough weight, you will probably be asked to check ketones and possibly increase carbohydrate intake.

Quick Reference on Amount of Carbohydrates Based on Total Calories

Calories	30%	40%	50%	60%
1,500	113 g	150 g	188 g	225 g
1,800	135 g	180 g	225 g	270 g
2,000	150 g	200 g	250 g	300 g
2,200	165 g	220 g	275 g	330 g
2,500	188 g	250 g	313 g	375 g

Source: Adapted from *Nutrition Therapy for Adults With Diabetes or Prediabetes: A Consensus Report.* American Diabetes Association. 2019.

Distribution & Timing of Meals

How you combine foods and the timing of meals will play a role in balancing your hunger and blood glucose. Spacing your meals and snacks 2–3 hours apart can ensure you don't become too hungry and, at the same time, prevent your blood glucose from going too high or too low. Some women might benefit from three meals and 1–3 snacks a day. A helpful tip is to combine a carb with a protein or fat in snacks to slow down the digestion of glucose. For example, a pita with hummus, an apple with peanut butter, or crackers with cheese. Check out more snack ideas in "Resources for All."

Keeping meals smaller throughout the day but adding snacks can also help prevent nausea or heartburn. Furthermore, the time of day can also affect how your blood glucose responds to carbohydrates. For example, hormones that cause insulin resistance might be higher in the morning, leading to more elevated blood glucose with breakfast.

Many women with diabetes will need to limit carbohydrates to 15–30 g at this time of day to minimize the peak after breakfast.

The best indicators of how an eating plan is working are your blood glucose and weight. In other words, if your blood glucose values are in target, and both you and your baby are gaining appropriate weight, then what you are doing is working! A glucose test should validate whichever meal planning tool you use. Let your finger checks be your guide! If you are under 120 mg/dL 2 hours after a meal and 90 mg/dL or less fasting, you are doing fantastic! Many women restrict themselves to eating just 15 g of carbs per meal, thinking this is what they *need* to do. In reality, they might be able to include more. This will all depend on your individual needs and postmeal checks.

Meal Planning & Carb Counting Methods

There are a number of methods that people with diabetes can use to plan healthy meals and manage blood glucose. It can be as simple as using your plate to guide appropriate portion sizes of different foods, or as complex as counting carbs in everything you eat. What works for you will depend on your health goals, your lifestyle, and your preferences. If you have a method that you have been successfully using, you can most likely stick with it during pregnancy. If there's room for improvement in your meal planning and blood glucose management, take this as an opportunity to explore new approaches and work with a dietitian or diabetes educator.

Diabetes Plate Method and Serving Sizes

The Diabetes Plate Method is an easy way to help you manage portion sizes and create a balanced plate. It emphasizes more vegetables and reduces foods with carbohydrates. It consists of visualizing a 9-inch plate and dividing it into three sections: Half of the plate is for nonstarchy vegetables (see list on pages 121 and 122), which are naturally low in carbohydrate and high in fiber and water. Divide the other half of the plate into two quarters. One-quarter of the plate should include a lean protein (4–5 oz) such as chicken, beef, low-mercury fish, turkey, or other protein; and the remaining one-quarter of the plate is for carbohydrate-rich foods like sweet potatoes, whole-grain pasta, brown rice, or legumes. This method is easy to follow and does not get into much detail about carb counting. Yet it also accounts for serving sizes by focusing more on nonstarchy vegetables. This method will always work, and it's simple to remember!

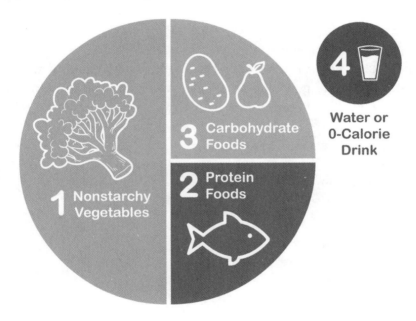

Key Points of the Diabetes Plate Method
- Fill 1/2 of your plate with nonstarchy vegetables.
- Fill 1/4 of your plate with carbohydrate-rich foods such as whole grains, fruits, starchy vegetables, low-fat yogurt/milk.
- Fill the remaining 1/4 with a lean protein.
- Include a small portion of healthy fat like avocado, olive oil, or nuts.
- Avoid sweetened beverages. Instead, drink water or non-caloric drinks.

Starchy Vegetables—Higher in carbohydrates. They are "carbohydrate foods" even though they are vegetables. Starchy vegetables include:

- Corn
- Potatoes
- Squash (Butternut, Winter, Acorn)
- Yam/Sweet Potatoes
- Peas
- Plantains

Nonstarchy Vegetables—Lower in carbs, usually higher in water content. They are good source of fiber, vitamins, and minerals. The following is a list of common nonstarchy vegetables:

- Amaranth or Chinese spinach
- Artichoke
- Artichoke hearts
- Asparagus
- Baby corn
- Bamboo shoots
- Beans (green, wax, Italian)
- Bean sprouts
- Beets
- Brussels sprouts
- Broccoli
- Cabbage (green, bok choy, Chinese)
- Carrots
- Cauliflower
- Celery
- Chayote
- Coleslaw (packaged, no dressing)
- Cucumber
- Daikon

- Eggplant
- Greens (collard, kale, mustard, turnip)
- Hearts of palm
- Jicama
- Kohlrabi
- Leeks
- Mushrooms
- Okra
- Onions
- Pea pods
- Peppers
- Radishes
- Rutabaga
- Salad greens (chicory, endive, escarole, lettuce, romaine, spinach, arugula, radicchio, watercress)
- Sprouts
- Squash (cushaw, summer, crookneck, spaghetti, zucchini)
- Sugar snap peas
- Swiss chard
- Tomato
- Turnips
- Water chestnuts
- Yard-long beans

Carb Counting

In diabetes management, counting carbs can be a great way to allow flexibility in what you eat and can help you manage your food and sugar intake. Carb counting is frequently done by people who use insulin, but you might have been told to start counting carbs in pregnancy to better manage your blood glucose. You can count carbs in different ways: reading labels, using a scale, or simply by understanding carbohydrate portions/choices. Make sure to read chapter 26, "How to Read a Nutrition Label," in the "Resources for All" section.

Using a Scale

A more advanced method of monitoring carbohydrates is to use a scale to determine the number of carbs per weight of a specific food. This method will be used mostly by women with type 1 diabetes or women with type 2 diabetes who are on insulin, as accurate carb counting will play a significant role in determining the correct dose of insulin to give.

Serving Sizes/Choices

A nutrition label will show you how many carbohydrates are in a food or serving size, yet many foods like fruits, veggies, and certain grains don't always have a label. What do you do then? This is when learning about servings/choices (or exchanges) comes in handy. The diabetes food choices are a list of seven different types of foods that are grouped and have similar amounts of carbohydrate, protein, and fat. One carbohydrate serving, or "choice," contains approximately 15 g carbohydrate. For example, one slice of bread equals 15 g carbohydrate, the same as one small apple (see table 10.1 on page 114 for more carb foods and their choice equivalents). The idea is that you can then exchange one serving of carbohydrate for another of your choice while keeping the amount of carbohydrate consistent. So, for example, if you were told to eat three servings of carbs in a meal, that would equal 45 g carbohydrates. Below are some standard carbohydrate servings. You can find out more about choices in the American Diabetes Association book, *Complete Guide to Carb Counting, 4th Edition*, which is available at ShopDiabetes.org.

Ways to Count Carbs

- Using the choice system, where one serving equals 15 g of carbs
- Reading nutrition label and focusing on total grams of carbs
- Using a foods scale
- A combination of all of the above

Examples of One Serving/Choice (About 15 g) of Carbohydrate

- 1 slice of whole-wheat bread
- 1/2 cup beans or lentils
- 1 cup milk
- 1/2 cup cooked oatmeal
- 1 cup berries/strawberries
- 1/2 whole-wheat pita bread
- 15 grapes
- 1 small apple
- 1/2 banana
- 1 small peach
- 1/2 cup corn or peas

Best Foods for You and Your Baby

As you might have guessed by now, there is no "pregnancy diet" or "eating for two." Instead, the same healthy and balanced eating habits that worked pre-pregnancy continue to apply. The main difference in pregnant women with diabetes is ensuring your blood glucose is in target. That said, the amount of carbohydrates in each meal, the type of carbs, and the timing and distribution of meals will be of great significance. A blood glucose test should validate whichever meal-planning tool you use. Let your finger checks be your guide. If you are under 120 mg/dL 2 hours after a meal and 90 mg/dL or less fasting, you are doing fantastic!

Consuming a wide variety of foods that include plenty of vegetables, slow carbs like whole grains, fruits, and healthy fats will make it easier for your baby to receive essential nutrients like folic acid, calcium, fiber, vitamin D, omega-3, DHA, and more. So, yay to all of those! Below you will find some of my recommendations for top foods to include in your diet, not only because of the high fiber intake, but also the unique nutrition profile they provide in pregnancy. These "diabetes pregnancy superfoods" will ensure your

TABLE 10.2 Best Foods to Include in Your Diet During Pregnancy

Food	Why it's so good
Salmon	Great source of essential omega-3, and high in vitamin D
Avocado	Healthy fat with omega-3 and lots of fiber, B vitamins, folate, and potassium
Sweet potatoes	High in fiber, vitamin A, and vitamin C; slow carb
Pistachios	High in nutrients, including fiber, fat, protein, potassium, and B vitamins
Eggs	Nutrient-packed, contains choline (25% of recommended daily intake), high in zinc and protein
Berries	High in vitamin C and fiber, rich in antioxidants; slow carb
Dark chocolate	Higher in fat and fiber and lower in sugar compared to milk chocolate, has polyphenols and flavonoids, which are antioxidants
Greek yogurt	Calcium, vitamin D, protein, and probiotics
Apples	High in fiber, vitamin C; slow carb
Nut butter	Healthy monounsaturated and polyunsaturated fats, high in fiber and protein
Dark leafy greens (spinach, kale, broccoli)	High in fiber, iron, calcium, folate, and potassium
Beans, lentils, legumes	Excellent source of plant-based protein, high in iron, folate, and calcium; slow carb
Sourdough or whole-wheat bread	Provides whole grains; slow carb
Quinoa	Whole grain, rich in fiber, B vitamins, and high in protein; slow carb

eating pattern is balanced, nutrient rich, and can prevent spikes in your blood glucose. There is an entire section dedicated to the essential nutrients you need during pregnancy in section 4, "Resources for All." In this section, you will find an in-depth discussion of special nutrients and supplementation like caffeine, folic acid, and non-nutritive sweeteners.

Key Takeaways from This Chapter

✓ The amount, type, timing and distribution of carbohydrates are all significant in managing your diabetes during pregnancy.

✓ You and your baby both need carbs as they serve as the body's preferred source of fuel. But you need to know *which ones* to eat, as well as *how many* and *when* to eat them.

✓ Chose SLOW CARBS! Choosing high-fiber, nutrient-dense carbs will help slow down the rise in high blood glucose.

✓ There are many methods you can use to plan healthy meals and manage blood glucose including the Diabetes Plate Method, counting carbs by reading nutrition labels, or using carb servings/choices.

REFERENCE
[1] Institute of Medicine. *Dietary Reference Intakes for Energy, Carbohydrate, Fiber, Fat, Fatty Acids, Cholesterol, Protein, and Amino Acids.* Washington, DC, The National Academies Press, 2005

CHAPTER 11

EATING OUT AND BEING SOCIAL

"I ate the same foods every day for 9 months."

—Said no one, ever!

Nothing beats the smell of fresh pizza dough coming out of the oven, topped with melted, salty cheese and homemade tomato sauce. Yes, I craved pizza while pregnant, but pizza was slightly more challenging to eat without experiencing higher blood glucose afterward. Before pregnancy, I would pride myself on being able to eat out and keep my blood glucose in target, and I assumed this skill would easily carry forward into pregnancy. After all, I'm a registered dietitian, and I know how to count carbs and choose the best foods while dining out, right? Wrong! Diabetes during pregnancy made it really challenging to eat out. It took many trials, errors, and modifications for me to feel comfortable eating outside my home. The struggle is real, but with the right tools, you will discover the joy of eating out without compromising your diabetes management.

You might have assumed that during pregnancy, eating out is off-limits, but you'd be surprised what a few useful tips can do! Being pregnant and having diabetes does not mean that you can't enjoy a night out with your friends and family. Because let's be real, nobody wants to eat the same foods every day. Dining out with friends when you live with diabetes and are expecting will require more preparation, but you will still be able to enjoy a meal without compromising your diabetes management. In this chapter, you will learn useful strategies on how to safely eat out when you have diabetes. We will provide you with tips when ordering at restaurants, discuss best restaurant foods, review healthy substitutions, and share ways to measure portion sizes. Having diabetes and living through two healthy pregnancies myself, I'm all about managing diabetes without sacrificing the love and joy this experience brings.

Why It Matters to Be Social

Eating out remains one of the hardest aspects to manage when you live with diabetes. It can be challenging to measure portion sizes, count carbohydrates, and resist the urge to order foods that might make your blood glucose higher than desired. Plus, you have little control over ingredients and preparation methods.

However, eating out is not just about the food—it's a social experience. We gather with friends, talk about life, and get to sit and relax. At times, living with diabetes can make you feel isolated because it can seem like you aren't allowed to enjoy the same foods as everyone else. Research shows that people with diabetes are twice as likely to suffer from depression compared to those without diabetes.[1,2] The additional demands of caring for your pregnancy on top of your diabetes add an extra layer of complexity. This is why caring for your emotional health is essential. Being pregnant and having diabetes should not stop you from socializing with friends and family. The more you educate your family members and the more you involve them in your diabetes care, the more supported you will feel.

Best Practices

To get started, here are some best practices to maximize your eating experience without derailing your diabetes care.

Before the Restaurant
- Try to go early. This way, you have time to take a walk in the evening if needed, and you are not starving when you get there.
- Look up the kind of cuisine, or even better, the menu. Doing a little research before, like knowing the type of food, will give you a better idea of what to expect. Plus, it can provide you with time to look up the carbs, if needed, or you might find that they have nutrition information labels.
- Make a reservation so you are not left waiting.

At the Restaurant
- If you know the portions are especially large, share with a friend or ask the waiter to split the plate beforehand and pack half of the dish in a doggy bag.
- Skip the bread basket.
- If you are taking insulin, aim to take your rapid-acting insulin 15–20 minutes before the meal arrives. This can be tricky, as restaurant timing is variable, but if your blood glucose is normal or slightly elevated, it will help avoid a spike afterward.
- Start with the veggies, soup, or protein first, then follow with the carbs. One small study showed that the order and timing in which you eat foods can affect blood glucose. Leaving carbohydrates for last may delay the rise in blood glucose,

so start with the veggies and leave the carbs for last. This way, you are getting satisfied with more fiber-rich, lower-carbohydrate foods.

After the Restaurant

- Bring a small piece of dark chocolate so you have a delicious alternative to a restaurant dessert on hand.(Did you know 1 square of dark chocolate has only 5 g of carbohydrate?) I did this many times, and it felt great to still indulge in something without overdoing it.
- Take a stroll afterward to help curb any blood glucose spikes. If you can walk to the restaurant, or even park toward the back of the parking lot even better! Every little bit counts. That little extra movement will also help prevent heartburn, which is more likely to occur as you progress into the second and third trimester and your uterus continues to expand.

Tips to Help You Master Your Ordering Technique

- Don't be afraid to ask for substitutions: *"Instead of the fries, can I get a salad?"*
- Healthy substitutions to consider: whole-wheat instead of white bread; brown rice instead of white rice; extra veggies instead of fries; dressing or cream on the side.
- *"Would you make sure to split the plate beforehand? I'll take the other half home with me."*
- Look for menu items that are boiled, steamed, grilled, or roasted.
- Ask to see the nutrition information. You may be surprised to find some restaurants offer a special menu with the nutrition information upon request— It doesn't hurt to ask!
- Avoid heavy sauces or creams, like alfredo sauce. Choose marinara or white wine sauces instead.
- Be mindful of hidden sources of sugar like barbecue sauces, honey dressings, and ketchup, and ask for the dipping sauce on the side.

Portion Sizes

Restaurants tend to serve large portions. One dish might be able to serve two to three people, so it will be vital for you to keep portions in check. Additionally, many restaurants don't have nutrition labels, which makes it harder to count carbohydrates. (Just remember to ask first!) Practicing your carb counting and monitoring portions at home using measuring cups, a scale, or household measurements is one of the best ways to prepare for counting carbs when eating out. This way, when you order a similar food at the restaurant, you'll be able to estimate carbs more accurately.

Tips for Keeping Portions and Carbs in Check

- Choose smaller-sized entrées like kid's portions or lunch-sized entrées.
- Split the entrée with your partner or have the server box half the meal ahead of time to take home.
- Use everyday visuals to help you estimate carbs:
  - One fist ≈ 1 cup
  - Palm of hand ≈ 3 ounces
  - Entire thumb ≈ 1 tablespoon
  - Tip of the thumb (to the first knuckle) ≈ 1 teaspoon

Recommendations for Common Restaurant Foods

Pizza—Go for thin crust and start with a salad. Top the pizza with plenty of nonstarchy veggies like mushrooms, artichokes, and peppers—they'll add extra fiber without having a big impact on your blood glucose. One slice of thin-crust pizza has about 20 g carbohydrate compared to 35 g for a regular pan crust.

Mexican—Beans, avocado, and salsa are all a YES! Add them to some grilled fajitas or in a Mexican burrito bowl (without the fried tortilla bowl, if it comes in one). Skip the tortilla chips and opt for whole-grain rice or bean soup. Beans, rice, and tortillas all have carbs, so try not to have them all in one meal. If you find it easy to go overboard with rice or flour tortillas, try beans and a corn tortilla to keep blood glucose steadier and portions in check.

Asian—Miso or hot soup makes a great starter (minimal calories or carbs and a lot of volume). For appetizers, skip the fried egg rolls; instead, choose edamame, a lower-carb nutrient powerhouse loaded with fiber and protein. Be careful with noodle dishes; they can be tricky because they are sometimes fried or prepared with heavy sauces. Sauces such as teriyaki, orange glaze, and BBQ can be a hidden source of added sugar, so be mindful when ordering. Ask for double the serving of veggies or select a protein dish like chicken stir-fry with extra vegetables and brown rice.

Italian—Skip the breadbasket and start with a tasty Italian classic: caprese salad (tomatoes and fresh mozzarella, all under 7 g of carbohydrate). It's often too tempting to order a pasta dish alone: consider splitting it, or opt for chicken or meat, and choose one side of carbs and veggies.

Burgers—Nowadays, most places allow you to order bunless burgers or use lettuce in place of a bun. If you are looking to reduce carbs, choose a bunless lettuce wrap or even half a bun. You can also swap the french fries for a salad and easily reduce the carb amount. If you see a veggie burger option, make sure you ask for the ingredients or nutrition information as some may have the same amount of carbs and saturated fat as a regular burger.

Key Takeaways from This Chapter

✓ Diabetes can often feel isolating. Don't let the anxiety of diabetes in pregnancy overwhelm you and stop you from socializing with friends and family. Instead, involve them in the process, and educate them on how certain foods affect your diabetes.

✓ When eating out in a restaurant, the more prepared you are, the better. Find out the type of food, look up the restaurant, and make an early reservation.

✓ Being pregnant and having diabetes does not mean you can't enjoy eating at your favorite restaurant, but it will require extra care and planning. Don't be afraid to speak up and ask for substitutions. Remember, if you are eating out, it's the restaurant's job to make it a pleasant experience.

REFERENCES

[1] Anderson R, Freedland K, Clouse R, Lustman P. The prevalence of comorbid depression in adults with diabetes. *Diabetes Care* Jun 2001; 24(6)1069–1078

[2] Egede, L. Diabetes, major depression, and functional disability among U.S. adults. *Diabetes Care* 2004; 27(2):421–428

EXERCISE AND STAYING ACTIVE

"If you start being active before pregnancy it's likely you'll continue it during pregnancy. This can make a big difference in how your body responds to insulin and will help avoid higher increases than would be normal in pregnancy."

—Jennifer Smith, RD, LD, CDCES, Director of Lifestyle and Nutrition at Integrated Diabetes Services. She has lived with type 1 diabetes for 32 years, is co-author of a book on pregnancy with type 1 diabetes, and is a mom of two healthy kids.

Yes, we all know exercise is good for us. But when it comes to diabetes and pregnancy, exercise can really make a big difference in your day-to-day diabetes management. Because pregnancy—regardless of diabetes—is an insulin-resistant state, anything you do to help lower the resistance will be of great benefit. Physical activity is known to benefit most women during pregnancy as it helps maintain a healthy weight, improves cardiovascular health, and reduces the risk of preeclampsia and cesarean delivery. For women with diabetes, regular physical activity, especially after meals, can help reduce postmeal blood glucose. When you are active, your body signals your muscles to utilize sugar more effectively and thus improves insulin sensitivity. Moreover, exercise helps you build the flexibility needed during labor and delivery, as well as the muscle tone that makes insulin work better. Think of exercise as a natural form of medication to lower blood glucose.

This chapter will discuss the importance of physical activity in pregnancy and give you guidance on which exercises are best and which to avoid. Remember, you don't need to run a marathon in order to see the benefits of physical activity: a simple 10- or 15-minute walk can help. Additionally, we'll discuss things to keep in mind when exercising, especially when it comes to experiencing low blood glucose. For even more information, make sure to check out chapter 4, "Maintaining a Healthy Weight and Staying Active during Pregnancy."

Benefits of Exercise

Nutrition, exercise, and medications are the three pillars for a healthy pregnancy. Being active during your pregnancy has numerous benefits: it increases strength; reduces complications; lowers blood glucose; lowers blood pressure; and prevents excess weight. Plus, it not only benefits you physically, but also mentally. Managing diabetes during pregnancy can be stressful, and engaging in regular physical activity can be a much-needed stress reliever and mood booster.

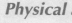

Physical and Mental Benefits of Exercise

- Helps maintain weight
- Helps prepare you for labor and delivery (shorter labor)
- Lowers blood pressure
- Aids in relieving constipation
- Helps posture
- Improves mood
- Reduces anxiety
- Helps you sleep better

Starting an Exercise Routine

The general recommendation during pregnancy is to engage in moderate exercise for 30 minutes every day or almost daily, according to guidance from the American College of Obstetricians and Gynecologists. If you have been working out prior to your pregnancy, there is no need to stop, but you might need to adjust the type of exercise, particularly in the last trimester of pregnancy (Table 12.1). For example, in the second and third trimesters, you should avoid exercises where you lie on your back, as this constricts blood flow to your baby. If you have not been active, then you should talk to your healthcare provider prior to starting an exercise routine. You might need to start slow and gradually build up endurance. Try to think of an activity that you *like* to do, rather than something you'll feel like you *have* to do. Finding the right type of activity for you will be important because you'll be more likely to stick with it. For me, it was walking, yoga, and lifting weights.

Best Timing and Types of Exercises during Pregnancy

Exercising first thing in the morning is a great way to start the day, or you can try to incorporate exercise after a snack or meal. But really, anytime that works for you is fantastic! Aerobic types of exercises like walking, cycling, swimming, and dancing will have a

TABLE 12.1 Recommended Exercises during Pregnancy

Exercises to include	Exercises to avoid
• Walking	• Contact sports, such as basketball, hockey, and football
• Yoga	
• Pilates	• Activities that involve jerky movements or high risk of falling, such as hiking, skiing, and aerobics
• Swimming	
• Light/moderate weightlifting	• Scuba diving
• Stationary bike	• Exercise at high altitudes
• Rowing	

greater impact on your blood glucose compared to anaerobic activities. Anaerobic exercises like strength training and weightlifting will not drop your blood glucose immediately, but they will be very helpful to include, as they help you build strength.

How to Fit in 30 Minutes of Exercise per Day in Real Life

Don't have time to go to the gym? No worries! Research shows breaking down 30 minutes into multiple 10- or 15-minute intervals can still provide you with health benefits.[1]

- Take the stairs on your way to work. (I walked up six flights of stairs up until week 38 of pregnancy.)
- After waking up, stretch and do some flexibility exercises.
- Download 15-minute guided exercises for pregnancy that use light to moderate weights.
- Take the dog for an extra walk.
- Try standing Pilates and/or barre-type exercises at home.
- Do a 15-minute set of supported pushups, squats, and planks.
- Take a short walk during your lunch break.
- Park your car farther away to squeeze in a short walk before and after work.
- Turn the music up and dance while doing house chores!

Considerations When Exercising

One of the most notable side effects when you are active is lower blood glucose. This will be welcome if you just ate; however, we don't want your blood glucose to fall too drastically. Start evaluating your blood glucose trends when you exercise. If it's possible for you to exercise around the same time each day, it will be easier to see the effects. In many cases, especially as your pregnancy progresses, you might not notice significant low blood glucose, but rather gradual drops that provide more stable blood glucose throughout the day.

TABLE 12.2 Symptoms of Low versus High Blood Glucose

Low blood glucose (hypoglycemia)	High blood glucose (hyperglycemia)
• Tremors/shakiness	• Tiredness
• Cold sweat	• Hunger
• Trouble concentrating	• Blurry vision
• Irritability	• Irritability

If you are noticing lower blood glucose when you exercise, you might require a small snack to keep you from going low. A snack with 15–30 g of carbohydrate might be enough, depending on the intensity and duration of the activity.

Keep in mind that if you are taking insulin, you are more susceptible to low blood glucose. Furthermore, the effects of exercise are not always immediate. (This is also known as the lag effect.) In fact, you might notice lower blood glucose as late as 6–8 hours after exercise. If you are using insulin and exercising later at night, keep in mind that you might require a bedtime snack in order to prevent you from going low while you sleep. (See Table 12.2 for some symptoms of low blood glucose.)

When Not to Exercise

- If blood glucose is >240 mg/dL and with ketones present
- If blood glucose is <70 mg/dL. (Treat blood glucose first until it normalizes.)
- If you have high blood pressure.
- If you are experiencing contractions.
- If you are experiencing shortness of breath.
- If you are experiencing dizziness.

TABLE 12.3 Best Foods or Drinks to Treat Low Blood Glucose— Examples of 15 g of Carbohydrate

Food	Carbohydrate (g)
3–4 glucose tabs	15
4–5 pieces of hard candy	15
4 oz juice	15
1 tablespoon honey	15

How to Treat Low Blood Glucose

Thinking of eating chocolate to treat low blood glucose? Think again! A chocolate bar will not be the best way to treat a low because the fat and protein in the chocolate will take much longer to reach your blood system. Use foods and drinks with easy-to-absorb carbohydrates, like juice, sugar, or glucose, and follow the 15–15 rule: 15 g of carbohydrate and recheck 15 minutes later. (See Table 12.3 for additional food recommendations to treat low blood glucose.)

Key Takeaways from This Chapter

✓ Exercise during pregnancy is safe and recommended. Aim for 30 minutes of daily activity.

✓ Exercise will help you lower blood glucose, improve strength, relieve stress, lower blood pressure, and maintain weight.

✓ Consider breaking up the exercise into 10- or 15-minute intervals. The key is to get moving!

✓ If you are using insulin, be aware that you might need to lower your dose or have a small snack if you are experiencing low blood glucose.

REFERENCE

[1] Thompson PD, Eijsvogels TMH. New physical activity guidelines: a call to activity for clinicians and patients. *JAMA* 2018;320(19):1983–1984

DELIVERY, BREASTFEEDING, AND THE FOURTH TRIMESTER

"Breastfeeding was very challenging, but also very rewarding. It helped me bond with my precious boys and improve my blood glucose and diabetes control."

—Emily Dudensing, registered dietitian diagnosed with gestational diabetes in all three of her pregnancies.

It's (almost) showtime! The long-awaited day is drawing near. The delivery and postpartum period are a critical time for both you and your baby. Maintaining blood glucose as close to target as possible throughout your pregnancy may help you avoid a C-section and increase the chances you deliver a full-term, healthy-weight baby. As you approach delivery, you will be closely monitored by your OB-GYN and perinatologist. They will be watching things like amniotic fluid, the baby's heartbeat, the size of the baby, breathing, fetal stress test, and (of course) your blood glucose. Remember, the last trimester is when your baby gains the most weight, which is why it's so important to keep a steady weight gain throughout pregnancy and avoid gaining too much weight in the first and second trimesters. In this chapter, we will cover what to expect at the time of labor and delivery. We will review delivery, postpartum care, and breast-feeding tips to help you nurse with confidence. Make sure to also read chapter 21, "The Birth—It's Go Time!", and chapter 6, "Delivery and the Future Ahead in Gestational Diabetes."

DID YOU KNOW? *Higher early morning and afternoon blood glucose levels in the second trimester, as well as higher evening blood glucose in the third trimester, are associated with a larger baby.[1,2]*

What to Expect During Labor and Delivery

Labor and delivery are a period of significant shifts in blood glucose, hormones, and insulin sensitivity. Most hospitals have set protocols for the management of women with diabetes during pregnancy that encompass mode of delivery, insulin management, blood glucose, medications, and more. As you approach your third trimester, you should make it a point to discuss them with your OB-GYN and become familiar with them. Ask about how they utilize pumps, sensors, insulin drips, treatment of low blood glucose in babies, formula, and so forth. Remember, you are your own advocate, so don't be afraid to speak up and develop a detailed postpartum plan with your team that meets your desires.

The guidelines for labor and delivery for women with diabetes recommend very tight blood glucose controls during this period: 72–126 mg/dL. Studies show that having higher blood glucose at the time of delivery increases the risk for your baby to have a low blood glucose at birth (neonatal hypoglycemia). If you are using insulin, many hospitals will want to place you on an insulin drip to control blood glucose and avoid hypoglycemia. If you are using a pump, you might be able to keep it, but you should discuss the details with your healthcare provider. (See more in chapter 21, "The Birth—It's Go Time!")

TABLE 13.1 Delivery Timing Guidelines for Women with Preexisting Diabetes

Diabetes Control	Complications	Delivery
Well controlled	None	39–40 weeks
Well controlled	Significant	37–39 weeks
Suboptimal	None	37–39 weeks
Suboptimal	Significant	34–39 weeks

Source: Adapted from Werner, E. *Medical Management of Diabetes Complicated by Pregnancy, 6th Edition.* American Diabetes Association. 2019.

Having tight control without the presence of vascular complications (e.g., high blood pressure, retinopathy, etc.) may allow you to have a safe delivery at full term (39–40 weeks). In the past, women with preexisting diabetes were told they needed to deliver by a specific week; however, advances in fetal testing have allowed for babies to be closely monitored and kept as close to term as possible if there are no signs of stress or complications (Table 13.1). In women with preexisting diabetes, the mode of delivery is determined on an

Questions to Ask Your Doctor/Healthcare Team in Preparation

- How will they determine the delivery date?
- Who will be managing your diabetes during labor?
- If you are having a C-section, what should you do the day you are scheduled to arrive at the hospital?
- If you are on insulin, will you take the same dose before your planned C-section?
- If you are wearing a pump or sensor, will you be able to keep them during labor?
- What is the treatment of low blood glucose if your baby were to experience it?
- Will you be able to nurse your baby if you are on diabetes medications?
- What will happen to your blood glucose after delivery?
- Will you need to continue your medications after giving birth?

individual basis, taking into account the clinical scenario. If you are well controlled with no sign of vascular complication, and the baby's at a healthy weight, you can be induced to deliver at 39 weeks. Having an induction at 39 weeks can increase the chances of vaginal delivery and decrease the chances of a C-section and shoulder dystocia. If, however, your baby's weight is estimated at greater than 4,500 g (9.9 lb), you will probably require a C-section.[3]

What to Expect Postpartum

Once the baby is born, the real work starts! The "fourth trimester" refers to the period from the moment your baby is born up until three months of age. This period is known for its many changes as both you and your baby adjust to this new life. Women with type 2 diabetes may return to pre-pregnancy oral antidiabetic medications or continue on insulin therapy, though don't be surprised if your insulin dosages are cut back drastically. One of the most significant changes you will notice is the sudden decrease in your need for insulin. If you are taking insulin, you will probably require half or one-third of the dose you were taking during pregnancy. Because the baby's placenta is gone, pregnancy-related insulin resistance drastically declines. If you had a C-section, proper diabetes management will be especially critical as it can take longer for your wound to heal. Expect to follow up with your healthcare provider 2 weeks after delivery and 6–8 weeks after that.

This period can also be a good time to talk to your provider about contraception and family planning. Planning pregnancy is critical in women with preexisting diabetes due to the need for tight blood glucose management before pregnancy to prevent congenital and birth malformations. Women with diabetes have the same contraception options and recommendations as those without diabetes. The biggest barrier for effective preconception planning is actually unplanned pregnancies. Because most pregnancies are unplanned, it's so important for women with diabetes to have family options reviewed regularly to make sure effective contraception is implemented. This also applies to women in the immediate postpartum period. Just because you recently had a baby does not prevent you from getting pregnant. And no, breastfeeding does not act as a safe contraception method (in case you were wondering)!

DID YOU KNOW? *Once you deliver your baby, your body will require less medication and register lower blood glucose levels. The change is almost instantaneous after your baby is born.*

Breastfeeding

"Can I breastfeed if I have diabetes?" Yes! The American College of Obstetrics and Gynecology HIGHLY recommends breastfeeding, as it's known to have many benefits for you and your baby. Breastfeeding will help you lose weight, improve insulin resistance, and boost your baby's immune system. Breast milk contains antibodies that protect your baby's immune system and reduce the risk of asthma, eczema, SIDS,[4] diabetes, celiac disease, and other allergic conditions. See Table 13.2 for additional benefits of breastfeeding for both you and your baby.

TABLE 13.2 Benefits of Breastfeeding

Benefits for your baby	Benefits for you
• Lowers the risk of allergic conditions (eczema, atopic dermatitis) • Promotes a healthy weight and lowers the risk of childhood obesity • Lowers the risk of diabetes, celiac disease, and infections • Boosts baby's immune system and strengthens gut bacteria	• Helps lose pre-pregnancy weight • Improves insulin resistance • Returns uterus to regular size and reduces postpartum bleeding • May lower the risk of breast and ovarian cancer • Saves money

Did you know you burn about 400 calories a day by breast-feeding? Yup, it's a lot of work! Be mindful that if you are breast-feeding, you are more prone to experience low blood glucose due to the extra demand for energy. So, if you are on medications, consider adjusting them to prevent hypoglycemia. You might also want to eat a carbohydrate snack before breastfeeding to keep your numbers from falling. See more ideas on breastfeeding snacks in section 4, "Resources for All."

Despite all of its known benefits, breastfeeding can be hard. For many women, it's not innate or natural in the first weeks. Plus, it can hurt, and it's emotionally and physically exhausting. But once you get the hang of it, it truly is a magical experience. For me, it wasn't easy initially, but thanks to the help of a lactation consultant, I knew what to expect and was able to do it for almost a year successfully. Successful breastfeeding will take practice, education, and determination. It's important to note that women with pre-existing diabetes are at increased risk for lactation complications like mastitis, reduced milk production, and candida infections compared to women who don't have diabetes; the rates for exclusively

Things to Consider when Breastfeeding

- Breastfeeding will lower your blood glucose, so make sure to have fast-acting carbohydrates at hand.
- Set juice boxes or create snack stations near the places you tend to breastfeed (next to your bed or by the rocking chair, for instance). That way, you are always prepared.
- Breastfeeding will make you hungry, so make sure to fuel up on wholesome, nutritious snacks, as your body is burning more calories. Have carbohydrate-containing snacks before and/or after breastfeeding.
- Stay hydrated. Drink one glass of water at every feeding.

breastfeeding in women with diabetes, primarily type 1 diabetes, are lower compared to mothers without diabetes.[5] Just know that if, for whatever reason, you decide not to breastfeed, that's okay, too. A growing and healthy baby is the most important thing. Below you will find some tips to prepare you and help you breastfeed with success.

Tips to Help You Breastfeed with Confidence and Success

- **Get informed.** Go to a breastfeeding class! This was the best thing we did. I got to know the myths, practiced positioning, and learned about latching. And many of these classes are free of cost at the hospital.
- **Don't wait to get help.** Find out if your hospital has a lactation consultant from day one.
- **Get to know hunger and fullness cues.** This will come with time and practice.
- **Make sure the baby is awake.** It might seem obvious, but this was a big lesson learned for me! This way, you make sure the baby gets a full feed. (I had to use a washcloth to wake up my first daughter.)
- **Trust!** This is the MOST important tip! You are not always in control. Trust your baby; trust in you. Trust you have *enough* breast milk. Trust your baby is eating what he or she needs.

Key Takeaways from This Chapter

✓ Keeping tight control on your blood glucose right up to delivery will help your baby have a healthy weight and a normal blood glucose, thereby avoiding infant hypoglycemia at birth (neonatal hypoglycemia).

✓ As you approach the last trimester, make sure you have a conversation with your healthcare team regarding the delivery protocol for women with preexisting diabetes. Don't be afraid to speak up and develop a detailed postpartum plan with your team that meets your desires.

✓ Expect to cut back your medication as your blood glucose will be lower. Your body will probably need less insulin immediately after your baby is born.

✓ Breastfeeding has many benefits for you (helps with weight loss, improves insulin resistance) and your baby (boosts immune system).

✓ Breastfeeding can also be challenging, so don't be afraid to seek the help of a lactation consultant, or better yet attend breastfeeding classes.

REFERENCES

[1] Draznin B (Ed.). *Diabetes Technology: Science and Practice.* Arlington, VA, American Diabetes Association, 2019

[2] Kerssen A, de Valk HW, Visser GH. Increased second trimester maternal glucose levels are related to extreme large-for-gestational age infants in women with type 1 diabetes mellitus. *Diabetes Care* 2007;30:1069–1074

[3] American College of Obstetricians and Gynecologists. ACOG practice bulletin no. 201: pregestational diabetes mellitus. *Obstet Gynecol* 2018; 132(6):e228–e248

[4] Hauck FR, Thomson JM, Tanabe KO, et al. Breastfeeding and reduced risk of sudden infant death syndrome: a meta-analysis. *Pediatrics* 2011; 128(1):103–1105

[5] Sparud-Lundin C, Wennergren M, Elfvin A, Berg M. Breastfeeding in women with type 1 diabetes: exploration of predictive factors. *Diabetes Care* 2011;34(2): 296–301

TYPE 1 DIABETES AND PREGNANCY

SECTION 3
Type 1 Diabetes and Pregnancy

Helpful Chapters to Review

- Chapter 4: Maintaining a Healthy Weight and Staying Active During Pregnancy
- Chapter 11: Eating Out and Being Social
- Chapter 12: Exercise and Staying Active
- Chapter 13: Delivery, Breastfeeding, and The Fourth Trimester

YOU CAN DO THIS!

"If you've decided to follow through with the pregnancy and become a mother, take a deep breath and brace yourself for one of the most challenging yet incredible experiences of your life. You are capable of so much more than you realize, and you can do this!"

—Ginger Vieira, author of "Pregnancy with Type 1 Diabetes," lives with type 1 diabetes and is a mom of two.

As a woman with type 1 diabetes, the idea of having a baby was terrifying to me. I had always heard horror stories of women with type 1 diabetes having all sorts of complications during pregnancy. (*Steel Magnolias*, anyone?) It took me several months—years, even—to feel like I was ready to start trying to have a family. And to this day, pregnancy with type 1 diabetes is one of the most challenging yet rewarding things I have ever done in my life. So, I truly understand what you are going through. Diabetes management during pregnancy is exceptionally demanding, but it's also *so* worth it! During those months, I learned a lot about being resilient, establishing discipline with my meals, and monitoring my blood glucose. But above all, I learned to be kind with myself and let go of things

I could not control. Now, I'm blessed to have two beautiful and healthy daughters, and I'm thankful I encountered no complications in my pregnancies. With the right support, careful planning, and dedication, you too will be able to have a successful pregnancy.

If you have been looking for a resource to help you navigate the ins and outs of pregnancy and type 1 diabetes, this is it! This section is for the woman who has type 1 diabetes and is seeking guidance on what to expect during each trimester of pregnancy, as well as practical solutions to the everyday challenges. You'll get real advice on everyday scenarios that will teach you *how* to manage your diabetes in the 9 months of your pregnancy. We will discuss real and effective strategies to get you ready for the time *you* decide is right. If you are already pregnant, no need to panic! You'll find advice to help you avoid the blood glucose rollercoaster ride and reach your pregnancy glucose targets. Additionally, we will discuss what to expect in each trimester and go over the use of pumps, sensors, and tech gadgets that could make your diabetes management more seamless. This section wraps up with postdelivery tips to get you ready for when the baby comes home, but make sure to read on to the next section, "Resources for All," where you will find ideas on snacks, essential nutrients for pregnancy, how to manage stress, "Q&A and Debunking Myths," and more. But first, let's talk about getting you ready for pregnancy.

chapter 15

PRECONCEPTION PLANNING AND GOALS

"Start to target pregnancy blood glucose before conception. Counseling should start before conception, if possible, to ensure every woman of childbearing age understands the basics of diabetes management in pregnancy."

—Jennifer Smith, RD, LD, CDCES, Director of Lifestyle and Nutrition at Integrated Diabetes Services. She has lived with type 1 diabetes for 32 years, is co-author of a book on pregnancy with type 1 diabetes, and is a mom of two healthy kids.

Preparing to have a child will take extra effort and preparation. It's important that you feel ready—or as ready as can be—to embark on this demanding period of care. Determining the "right time" to have a baby will be a personal decision, but one thing is clear: having your diabetes in tight and stable control *before* pregnancy is vital in ensuring a healthy pregnancy. Research clearly shows that having an A1C as close to target as possible (under 6.5%) and keeping blood glucose in optimal range before you become pregnant is a game changer when it comes to preventing malformations in babies.

The most critical time for your baby is the period from days 14–56 after conception. During this time, your baby's organs are being formed (lungs, heart, brain, ears, and so forth). Birth defects like heart problems and neural tube defects may occur when the fetus is exposed to consistently high blood glucose levels early in pregnancy. Keep in mind that a sporadic high blood glucose reading is not a major issue; rather, it's consistently higher blood glucose levels that put your baby at risk. If you are unable to reach blood glucose targets or if you have an A1C above 6.5%, you might be advised by your healthcare team to hold off pregnancy until you attain tighter control of blood glucose. That's how important it is. On the flipside, studies also show that receiving the appropriate care and education (preconception planning) significantly reduces the risk of any birth defects. So, the more prepared and informed you are, the better for you and your baby.

In this chapter, we will discuss glucose goals before and during pregnancy and some important tests to have before pregnancy. We'll review the pregnancy team and explore how to fine-tune insulin doses. Last, we will highlight the golden rules of nutrition and physical activity that will prepare you for what's ahead. The goal of this chapter is to give you the tools you need to feel equipped and ready to embark on a healthy pregnancy.

What this chapter will cover:
- Blood glucose targets before and during pregnancy
- Getting to know your pregnancy team
- Tests to get done before pregnancy
- Understanding how to fine-tune insulin dosages
- Golden rules of wholesome nutrition and exercise

Blood Glucose Goals and Why Pregnancy Planning Matters

As you know (since you live with type 1 diabetes), keeping your blood glucose in control is essential to help keep you healthy and avoid long-term complications. However, you might not know that during pregnancy, glucose targets are tighter compared to nonpregnancy. The American Diabetes Association and other major institutions recommend fasting blood glucose of <95 mg/dL and either <140 mg/dL 1 hour after meals or <120 mg/dL 2 hours after meals, along with an A1C of 6.5% or under without significant hypoglycemia.

Yup, I know what you're thinking: blood glucose under 140 mg/dL at *all* times and waking up below 95 mg/dL? Impossible! And trust me, I felt the same way. For many women with type 1 diabetes, these new targets can seem intimidating and, frankly, impossible to achieve. Waking up with blood glucose under 95 mg/dL can be scary, especially if you have an impaired ability to detect low blood glucose (also known as hypoglycemia unawareness). To give you a little perspective, fasting blood glucose during pregnancy in women without diabetes is around 60–70 mg/dL. This range is considered normal and healthy for pregnant women. However, for the pregnant woman with preexisting diabetes, this would be considered a low blood glucose reading. This is just the first of many reasons why diabetes during pregnancy is an entirely different ballgame! But remember, the goal during pregnancy is still to keep your blood glucose as close to normal as possible without enduring hypoglycemia; you just have to redefine "normal" (Table 15.1).

DID YOU KNOW?

Blood glucose goals in pregnancy are much tighter than what you might be used to. For some women with diabetes, having a fasting blood glucose of 95 mg/dL can be considered low, but in pregnancy this is optimal.

TABLE 15.1 Blood Glucose Goals, Pregnancy vs. Nonpregnancy

	Pregnancy	Nonpregnancy
Fasting	<95 mg/dL	80–130 mg/dL
1 hour after meals	<140 mg/dL	<180 mg/dL
2 hours after meals	<120 mg/dL	<180 mg/dL
A1C	Under 6.5%	<7.0%

Source: Standards of Medical Care in Diabetes–2020. American Diabetes Association.

When you live with diabetes, it will be especially important to make sure your blood glucose values are in check before getting pregnant, because the first 3 months are critical in your baby's development. The first 8–10 weeks after conception are the most vital for your baby because this is when organs are formed (organogenesis). As pregnancy progresses, it will become more challenging to manage your blood glucose, so it's important to get off to a good start and get used to these new blood glucose norms early on. If you are experiencing frequent lows, your targets might need to be adjusted and individualized with your medical team. If you are having trouble meeting these new pregnancy blood glucose goals, don't get frustrated. It might take time and require tweaks in your diabetes management. In the next chapter, "Strategies to Avoid Spikes in Blood Glucose," you'll learn about practical actions you can take to start getting ready for pregnancy and avoid spikes or drops in blood glucose targets. These tactics can also be incorporated throughout your pregnancy and will help you maintain blood glucose goals.

Topics to Cover at Your Diabetes Prenatal Education Visit

- Pregnancy blood glucose goals.
- Monitoring goals for pregnancy.
- Medications to avoid during pregnancy due to possible birth defects (ACE inhibitors, statins, angiotensin receptor blockers).
- What to do when blood glucose levels are high/low.
- Carb counting, understanding insulin-to-carb ratios, correction factors, and targets.
- Insulin management review.
- Nutrient recommendations/important nutrients (folic acid, DHA, calcium, choline, and others).
- Checking for ketones. (When and where?)
- Food, insulin, and blood glucose logs.
- Meal plan review. (Food safety and evaluation of weight gain recommendations and monitoring.)

The Diabetes and Pregnancy Team

They say it takes a village to raise a child. The same can be said for managing diabetes in pregnancy. It takes a team approach to help you achieve tight blood glucose control and support you along these 9 months. Be prepared to have multiple appointments during this time, especially as you approach the last trimester. You might be visiting your OB-GYN and maternal-fetal medicine specialist or perinatologist twice a week starting at week 30, so make sure you get acquainted with them. You might not have access to all of these healthcare providers. Many places across the U.S. lack a multidisciplinary team focused solely on diabetes and pregnancy. If you find a hospital that includes all the disciplines, you are in luck.

But don't worry, you can always build your team and make it work for you. Let's first discuss who they are.

- **Endocrinologist**—A medical doctor specialized in treating diabetes and other endocrine disorders. If you are living with diabetes, you probably see an endocrinologist every 6–12 months. An endocrinologist is an integral team member as they are the diabetes "gurus" and will be monitoring your insulin regimen, labs, and diabetes control throughout your pregnancy. Make sure you pick one that is familiar with your needs.
- **Obstetrician**—Your OB-GYN is the "pregnancy doctor" who you will see very frequently. They will be the ones to actually deliver your baby and keep a close eye on ensuring that your baby is growing and thriving accordingly. When choosing an OB-GYN, you might want to ask what type of experience they have with women with diabetes. Ask about the labor and delivery process and how they usually manage women with diabetes in pregnancy. Make sure you feel comfortable asking questions and being honest with them, as you will see your OB-GYN every week near the end of your pregnancy.
- **Maternal-fetal medicine specialist (MFM)**—A doctor specializing in high-risk pregnancies, also known as a perinatologist. Many OB-GYNs don't work with high-risk pregnancy clients like women with diabetes, but instead refer them to an MFM. An MFM is highly specialized in managing high-risk pregnancies, including gestational diabetes and preexisting diabetes. They will be doing more complex anatomy checks, assessing amniotic fluid, and performing fetal sonograms, among other exams. Depending on where you go, an MFM will see you weekly instead of your OB-GYN or endocrinologist.
- **Certified diabetes care and education specialist (CDCES or CDE)**—A diabetes care and education specialist is a person specialized in giving you the tools you need to thrive with

your diabetes. They will provide diabetes-specific education to make managing diabetes easier. It can be a nurse educator, dietitian, nurse practitioner, or other trained professional. Make sure the CDCES you are seeing is experienced in working with pregnant women. In many offices, the nurse educator or CDCES will be the one closely following your blood glucose throughout pregnancy.

- **Registered dietitian (RD/RDN)** — The nutrition expert responsible for answering all your nutrition questions. It will be beneficial to meet with a dietitian before, during, and even after your pregnancy to review things like essential nutrients, the timing of meals and snacks, assistance with nausea, meal planning, carb counting, and more. If your doctor's office does not have one, you can find one by visiting www.eatright.org/find-an-expert.
- **Ophthalmologist** — A doctor that specializes in the study and treatment of the eye. Because pregnancy increases pressure to the eyes, you are at a higher risk of developing retinopathy. Make sure you visit the ophthalmologist to get a dilated eye exam before pregnancy and 3 months into your pregnancy to assess any changes.
- **Partner/significant other** — Yes, your partner will be a crucial player in this journey! It might seem obvious, but getting your partner involved early on in the pregnancy process is very important. If you're used to managing your diabetes on your own, your partner may not know the intricacies involved in diabetes care. Bring them along to the diabetes educator visit and teach them to check your blood glucose. It will be a good idea for them to know your signs and symptoms of low blood glucose. (See my partner's story later in this chapter.)
- **Social worker** — A mental health professional who can help you navigate any financial, social, and psychological health needs. They can help you get the support you need, including

locating a counselor or helping you navigate through your insurance so that you understand what is covered.

- **Lactation consultant**—A professional breastfeeding specialist that will help you breastfeed your baby successfully and support you if you experience difficulties. Some hospitals have lactation consultants on their services so you can ask to see one on your fist day after labor and delivery. You could also take breastfeeding classes beforehand to prepare you for what to expect.

My Partner's Story

As we were preparing for pregnancy, I had my husband wear a demo insulin pump for a few days to experience a bit of what life is like for a person with diabetes. I wanted him to put himself in my shoes and experience what I go through on a daily basis. He didn't last 2 days. All the same, it really helped him understand the complexities and daily tasks of keeping up with my diabetes. The main lesson: It's hard for people, even your closest friends and family, to understand what it means to live with diabetes. Allow them to be part of it by teaching them how to check blood glucose, how to understand low and high blood glucose symptoms, and what to do in case of emergency.

Pre-Pregnancy Tests

Before pregnancy, your medical team might want to check specific labs to make sure everything is in order before pregnancy. These might include the following:

- Thyroid test
- A1C
- Iron
- Vitamin D
- Dilated eye exam
- Blood pressure
- Assessment of cardiac health and kidney problems

Pre-Planning Appointment Checklist

☐ **Visit endocrinologist.** Discuss preconception blood glucose goals, review medications, get thyroid exam, screen for kidney disease, and obtain urine samples.

☐ **A1C under 6.5%.** The goal is to have A1C as close to normal and under 6.5% without the presence of low blood glucose.

☐ **Ophthalmologist exam with retina dilation.** Dilated eye examinations should occur ideally before pregnancy or in the first trimester, and then patients should be monitored every trimester and for 1 year postpartum, as indicated by the degree of retinopathy and as recommended.

☐ **Dentist appointment.** The physiological changes during pregnancy put women at risk for dental problems such as cavities, gingivitis, and plaque. If you have diabetes, it will be important for you to visit your dentist for routine checkups.

☐ **Keep and maintain blood pressure goals (<130/80 mmHg).** If you have high blood pressure, make sure to talk to your doctor about which medications are safe to use. (No ACE inhibitors.)

☐ **Take a prenatal vitamin with folic acid.** Begin taking at least 3 months before pregnancy.

☐ **Visit with CDCES and RD/RDN.** Discuss current medication and lifestyle treatment, evaluate patterns and trends, review important nutrients, discuss strategies for keeping blood glucose in target.

Preconception Checklist

Education	❏ Nutrition assessment for
	   ● Underweight or overweight
	   ● Meal planning
	   ● Important nutrients during pregnancy
	   ● Caffeine intake
	   ● Safe food practices
	❏ Counseling on diabetes and pregnancy
	   ● Natural history of insulin resistance and increased need for insulin during pregnancy
	   ● Preconception targets
	   ● Avoidance of low blood glucose
	   ● Avoidance of high blood glucose/DKA
	   ● Labor and delivery
	❏ Lifestyle recommendations for
	   ● Exercise
	   ● Stress management
	   ● Sleep
	❏ Supplementation
	   ● Folic acid and prenatal vitamins
	   ● Over-the-counter medications

Medical assessment	❏ Review current medications (avoid ACE inhibitors, angiotensin receptor blockers , statins) ❏ General evaluation of overall health ❏ Evaluate for diabetes complications, including hypoglycemia unawareness, DKA, high blood pressure, retinopathy
Screening	❏ Diabetes complications, including foot exam, thyroid function, kidney function, cardiac risk factors, and more ❏ Anemia ❏ Genetic carrier for other conditions
Immunization	❏ Rubella ❏ Varicella ❏ Hepatitis B ❏ Influenza

Source: Adapted from *Standards of Medical Care in Diabetes–2020*. American Diabetes Association.

Wholesome Nutrition and Staying Active

You've heard it before: Proper nutrition, staying active, and medications are the cornerstones of diabetes management. (I might add a fourth one, emotional health, which is critical when you live with this condition 24/7.) Understanding how to count carbohydrates accurately as well as knowing how different foods affect your blood glucose prior to pregnancy will be fundamental in your pre-pregnancy planning. Following a balanced and healthy eating plan will be important for a few key reasons. First, it will be easier to maintain a healthy weight and manage your blood glucose. And second, a healthy eating plan will promote your baby's growth and development.

There is no such thing as a "diabetes diet." Instead, there are many healthful eating patterns you can adopt. Keep in mind, diabetes is very individualized, and different people can react to food in different ways. My body's blood glucose reaction to pasta can be very different to yours! Nevertheless, the more accustomed you are to eating healthy meals and snacks prior to becoming pregnant, the less stressful it will be during pregnancy. Meeting with a registered dietitian can guide you in making better choices for your diabetes and creating an individualized plan that works for your needs. We'll dive a little deeper into this topic in the next chapter, where you will find golden rules to live by to avoid spikes in blood glucose during pregnancy. Additionally, make sure to read section 4, "Resources for All," chapters 24, 25, and 28.

What to Cover during Nutrition Visit Preconception Planning

- Carb-counting skills
- Micronutrient needs and carbohydrate timing
- Strategies to maintain a healthy weight
- Strategies to avoid spikes in blood glucose
- Impact of exercise
- Effects of food/digestion on blood glucose
- Timing of insulin
- Advanced food bolus

Key Takeaways from This Chapter

✓ Preconception planning is vital in helping you fine-tune diabetes self-management skills and get your ready to embark this journey.

✓ Aim to have an A1C as close to target and under <6.5% before pregnancy.

✓ Blood glucose targets are tighter in pregnancy compared to non-pregnancy: Fasting <95mg/dL, 1 hr < 140mg/dL, 2 hr <120mg/dL.

✓ Preplanning is key! The first trimester in pregnancy (8–10weeks) is the most important for your baby's formation, so ensuring your blood glucose is in target range will help prevent malformations. Keep in mind, one high blood glucose will not put your baby at risk: It's consistent high blood glucose that matters.

✓ Expect to get various tests as part of the medical assessment and screening to ensure everything is in order before pregnancy.

✓ Meet with a registered dietitian and diabetes care specialist for a prenatal appointment to fine-tune your carb-counting skills, review important nutrients during pregnancy, and create a plan that works for your needs.

STRATEGIES TO AVOID SPIKES IN BLOOD GLUCOSE

"A day of elevated blood sugars is like giving your baby an occasional candy bar; one time is okay, but if you give one every day, it becomes a problem."

—Carlos Garcia, OB-GYN, Miami, FL.

By definition, type 1 diabetes means your body does not produce insulin. Therefore, it is unable to normalize blood glucose after ingesting carbs—this is where diabetes self-management skills come into play. Our job (as individuals with type 1 diabetes) is to be our artificial pancreas and ensure blood glucose spikes don't happen. But it's impossible to have "perfect blood glucose 24/7" because we're not a real pancreas. I've always considered myself to be under good control, and yes, I am a diabetes educator, but even for me, these targets seemed almost unattainable. I remember when I first learned that I should aim for a blood glucose of 120mg/dL one hour after eating. In my head, I just thought, *How on earth do I get blood glucose under 120mg/dL if I just ate—and I'm supposed to maintain this for 9 months?* It just seemed impossible. Ensuring you maintain blood glucose from spiking after meals will require additional training and practicing, but hopefully, after reading this section you will feel confident you can do this.

This chapter will highlight practical strategies you can implement in your diabetes routine to help avoid the rollercoaster highs and lows that frequently come in tight glucose management. You might already be using some of them in your everyday self-care routine, but these strategies will be particularly helpful throughout the entire pregnancy. They are what I like to call the "golden rules of diabetes," and the earlier you start to incorporate these practices and make them a habit, the more natural they will become as your pregnancy progresses. Please remember that these are just tips to help your diabetes management become easier. I used all of these strategies and still continue to live by some of them. Nevertheless, it will be very important to consult with your medical team before making any adjustments to your insulin dosages.

Golden Rules of Diabetes

- **Strategize the order of the meal. Start with veggies first and leave the carbs for last.** If you start a meal with your veggies first, followed by protein and then carbs, the insulin will have more time to act in your system because carbohydrates will be eaten last. Leaving carbohydrates for last may delay the rise in blood glucose, and one small study showed that the order and timing in which you eat foods can affect blood glucose. Additionally, starting with the veggies first can help you fill up with lots of fiber-rich veggies, which are lower in carbohydrates, and can reduce hunger.
- **Pre-bolus.** Taking insulin before meals, or pre-bolusing, is as important as knowing how to count carbs correctly. For me, it was a revelation. It will truly make the difference between a blood glucose of 160 mg/dL after lunch or a 110 mg/dL 2 hours later. Remember, insulin takes about 30+ minutes to start acting, and during pregnancy, this might take even

longer due to hormones and delayed gastric absorption. At the end of the third trimester, you might need to take insulin about 30–45 minutes before meals (especially breakfast) to maintain blood glucose in target 2 hours later. Pre-bolusing can be very, very frightening if you are not used to taking insulin before meals. Getting used to pre-bolusing while you are planning for pregnancy will prepare you for doing it when you are pregnant, and you will see the difference it makes.

> **TIP:** *If you are eating out and don't know when food will arrive, you can take half of the insulin dose before and the other half when the food gets there. This way, you avoid the risk of hypoglycemia at the restaurant in case the food takes longer.*

- **Focus on Choosing Slow Carbs.** We know carbohydrates raise blood glucose, but not all carbs are created equal nor do they have the same effect on your blood glucose (as you might already noticed) When choosing carbohydrates, choose what I call "slow carbohydrates". This is not a scientific term, but one I like to use for carbohydrates that are both high in fiber and nutrient dense. These type of carbs will fill you up and provide you the necessary vitamins and minerals, but will be slower to raise your blood glucose. Slow carbs include whole grains, fruits with plenty of fiber and legumes, such as lentils or beans, which include protein, and can help curb spikes in blood glucose. Eating foods high in fiber can slow down the absorption of glucose into the bloodstream because fiber is not fully broken down and digested. Foods with fiber take longer to raise your blood glucose, and therefore prevent sharp spikes in blood glucose (more on fiber below). Carbs that contain protein, like legumes, pulses, and even sprouted bread, can also be considered slow carbs because they will raise blood glucose much more slowly than highly processed foods made with white flour, like pretzels, white rice, and others. But keep in mind that there are individual variations on how certain foods affect you, so no two people with diabetes are the same. If you noticed certain foods impacted you differently pre-pregnancy, keep that in mind especially if it was working for you. The main point is to choose your carbs wisely, not deprive yourself of them. See a detailed list in chapter 9, "Everything you Need to Know about Nutrition during Pregnancy and Type 2 Diabetes."

- **Add fat/protein to meals.** Similar to eating slow carbs, including fats and protein to a meal will slow down how glucose is absorbed. Including them is a way of decreasing the glycemic index of foods. Plus, they will keep you feeling fuller for longer. Make sure you add healthy fats like nuts, avocado, olive oil, or olives. Choosing snacks that contain fats and protein may also help curve a spike in blood glucose, especially if you need to cover it with insulin. (See more on snacks in the next section, "Resources for All.")

- **Avoid overtreating lows.** When you were first diagnosed with diabetes, you were told to treat blood glucose with the 15–15 rule. Sound familiar? Fifteen grams of fast-acting carbohydrate and waiting 15 minutes to retest (Table 16.2). Or you might be used to using a low blood glucose to indulge in your favorite ice cream. Well, in pregnancy, this rule will not necessarily apply. You may only need 5–10 g carbohydrate to treat low blood glucose depending on how low it is. If your blood glucose is 73 mg/dL versus 50 mg/dL, this will make a difference in the amount of carbohydrates you use to treat it. Remember, a low can be very dangerous for you because you run the risk of passing out or falling.

> **TIP:** *In pregnancy, it is so much easier to treat a low blood glucose than to manage high blood glucose. With a low, you eat 5–15 g of carbs and wait 15 minutes. With high blood glucose, you need to take insulin, and it might take up to 2 hours for your blood glucose to come to target.*

TABLE 16.1 **Best Foods or Drinks to Treat Low Blood Glucose with 15 g of Carbs**

Food	Carbohydrate (g)
3–4 glucose tabs	15
4–5 pieces of hard candy	15
4 oz juice	15
1 tablespoon honey	15

- **Mind the timing of the meal (breakfast versus lunch versus dinner).** During pregnancy, morning blood glucose can be harder to manage due to the influx of hormones and the insulin resistance that naturally occurs at this time of day. Knowing this, you may choose to modify the number of carbs eaten at breakfast to 15–25 g. As you move along into the last trimester, you will become more insulin resistant in the morning and may only tolerate 15 g of carbs. By keeping the carb amounts lower in the morning and higher as the day progresses, you still get enough carbs, but redistribute them based on timing.[1]
- **Split the meal.** If you eat a large amount of carbs, you will start noticing higher peaks, especially 1–2 hours afterward. Splitting the meal can help counteract the spikes in blood glucose that are more likely to occur when eating the whole meal at once. You would still take your entire insulin dose for the meal, but eat just half of the meal; then, you eat the other half about 1–2 hours later. Remember, pregnancy hormones make it harder for you to process insulin after meals by creating additional resistance and making insulin act the opposite of how it usually works (raising blood glucose versus decreasing blood glucose). As a result, you may find insulin does not work as fast as before, creating spikes in blood glucose.

- **Consider a super bolus (for insulin pump users only).**
A "super bolus," a term coined by Dr. John T. Walsh, refers to a type of insulin delivery bolus that drops insulin from the basal rate and adds it on top of your meal or correction bolus. This, in essence, borrows insulin from the basal and gives more insulin up front where it is needed the most. For example, if your basal rate is 1.2 units per hour, you could give this additional 1.2 units on top of your meal/correction bolus and decrease your basal rate by 80–90% for the next 3 hours. A super bolus will decrease blood glucose faster than a traditional insulin bolus, so this strategy could be helpful when eating high-glycemic foods, large amounts of carbs, or in the morning.

Key Takeaways from This Chapter

✓ Maintaining blood glucose under tight control will take practice and fine-tuning.

✓ The earlier you can feel confident using these techniques before pregnancy, the more natural it can feel during pregnancy.

✓ Taking insulin before meals, or pre-bolusing, was one the most important strategies I used. Consider pre-bolusing at least 15–20 min before meals. This may need to be done earlier as the pregnancy progresses.

✓ Breakfast may be the most challenging meal due to insulin resistance and pregnancy hormones. Consider modifying carbs to 15–30 g for breakfast.

✓ Be mindful when treating lows, depending on how low your blood glucose is. You may only need 5–10 g carbohydrate to treat low blood glucose. But always make sure you have a fast-acting carb at hand.

REFERENCE
[1] American Diabetes Association. 14. Management of diabetes in pregnancy: *Standards of Medical Care in Diabetes—2019. Diabetes Care* 2019;42(Suppl. 1): S165–S172

DIABETES TECHNOLOGY— PUMPS, SENSORS, AND MORE

"I had the misconception that you needed to use an insulin pump during pregnancy—which is not true. Realize that you need to do what works for you and there is no ONE best tool for everyone. I used multiple daily injections for both of my pregnancies, along with a sensor, and I was able to have a healthy pregnancy and keep my A1C in the 5–6% range."

—Ginger Vieira, author of "Pregnancy with Type 1 Diabetes," lives with type 1 diabetes and is a mom of two.

Let's talk technology. There is no question that it has improved the lives of people with diabetes, but for some people, embracing technology can be hard, especially if you've been managing your diabetes in the same way for many years. For me, using a continuous glucose monitor (CGM) during both of my pregnancies was life changing. It allowed me to view my blood glucose at all times, and because of it, I was able to make better choices and adjust as needed.

In this chapter, we will review the different types of insulin pumps and CGMs (also known as sensors) and discuss the pros and cons of using them in pregnancy. Additionally, we will highlight the best time to start using them. Both pumps and sensors have the potential to improve quality of life, reduce hypoglycemia, and allow for more flexibility in lessening the burden of diabetes. There is no *single* best technology tool for diabetes. The key is identifying the technology that fits and works for you. So, let's first understand what pumps and sensors do, and then how they can help you make diabetes more manageable.

Insulin Pumps

Insulin pumps have been around for more than 40 years and are more commonly used in people with type 1 diabetes versus type 2. Insulin pumps provide a better way of delivering insulin since they mimic the body's physiological method of supplying insulin. A pump is a programmable device (think of it as a calculator) that provides rapid-acting insulin in very small, pulse-like dosages, also referred to as basal rates, similar to how your pancreas releases insulin. An insulin pump provides greater flexibility because you can customize the basal rates at a given time. You can also time the insulin bolus based on the food you eat and take insulin without the need for an additional injection. (Yay for fewer injections!)

The flexibility for insulin dosing and bolus calculations can be especially appealing in pregnancy since the amount of insulin required during the day versus the night is very different due to pregnancy hormones. Insulin pump therapy has been shown to improve blood glucose variation, improve A1C, and reduce hypoglycemia in individuals with either type 1 or type 2 diabetes.[1] However, studies show no significant differences in pregnancy outcomes or diabetes management in pregnant women who used multiple insulin injections versus an insulin pump.[2,3,4] It's worth noting that the studies did not reflect the newest insulin pumps on the market, which have improved usability and accuracy. Regardless, if you are using insulin injections and you feel comfortable with that approach, it is perfectly fine.

Another critical factor to consider is the timing of initiating use of an insulin pump. Ideally, an insulin pump should be started pre-pregnancy to allow you enough time to become familiarized with the device, understand dosages, and establish the right amounts before pregnancy. If you are new to a pump, expect to have comprehensive training to discuss troubleshooting and advanced features. Some potential adverse effects of wearing a pump include diabetic ketoacidosis (DKA) and severe hypoglycemia (although they are not so common). When you use a pump, a site malfunction will lead to a faster onset of DKA; therefore, expect to change your insulin pump site every 2 days rather than 3 to prevent any site issues. (See Table 17.1 for a comparison of the pros and cons of using an insulin pump.)

TABLE 17.1 Pros and Cons of Using an Insulin Pump in Pregnancy

Pros	Cons
• More flexibility to deliver insulin.	• Can lead to faster onset of DKA due to potential site issues.
• Can tailor basal insulin to match rise in blood glucose due to hormones.	• Higher cost if not covered by insurance.
• Less need for calculation and math. (You can set multiple insulin-to-carb ratios, and it will calculate instant carb correction and insulin-on-board amounts.)	• Requires training and a learning curve once started.
• Advanced features like temporary basal, insulin on board, and bolus rates that can make it easier to make insulin adjustments.	• Requires psychological readiness to be connected to a device.

The bottom line: An insulin pump is a safe and convenient option in pregnancy, though not necessarily more so than multiple insulin injections. As I always say, the pump is only as good as the user. It comes down to individual proficiency in using both injections and an insulin pump. Both methods are effective ways of managing diabetes in pregnancy. The most important aspect is that you feel comfortable in the treatment modality used, and you can troubleshoot accordingly.

A Deep Dive to Understanding Your Insulin Pump Features

- **Basal rate**—Pumps provide continuous insulin delivery via small, pulse-like doses of rapid-acting insulin given every hour that replace the long-acting insulin you take. For example, if you currently take 30 units of long-acting insulin at night, divide 30 units by 24 (24 hours in a day) to get the hourly basal rate, which would come out to 1.25 units per hour. Basal rates are usually 50% of total insulin dose, and the remainder is from bolus or food insulin. However, in pregnancy, it is not unusual to see basals in the 30%–40% range with the remainder dose for food boluses.

- **Bolus/insulin-to-carb ratio**—This value represents how much insulin is needed to cover a certain amount of carbohydrates. For example, you might require 1 unit of insulin for every 10 g of carbohydrates. This figure is very individualized and, again, will depend on the time of day. It's not unusual for people with diabetes to have different ratios throughout the day. An insulin pump allows for different ratios to be set at different times, which can help match the rise in hormones and blood glucose. In pregnancy, the morning ratio will usually be "stronger" compared to other times of the day due to increased insulin resistance during this time. As your pregnancy progresses, expect your ratios to be higher (i.e., lower numbers), so that by the third trimester you might require 1 unit for only 3 g of carbohydrates (Thank you, pregnancy hormones!) Human placental lactogen will impact postmeal values in particular, which is why more insulin is needed to cover for the same amounts of carbohydrates.[5]

- **Blood glucose correction/insulin sensitivity factor—** This represents how much insulin is needed to bring your blood glucose to target. Just like carb ratios, correction factors are individualized and calculated based on your total daily insulin dose. An insulin pump allows for different corrections to be set at different times of the day. For example, 1 unit of insulin will drop you 45 points but this might be different at night. During pregnancy, your corrections will need to be changed as your body will require more insulin.

- **Insulin duration—** This is a measure of how long the rapid-acting insulin will work. Most pumps have this setting set at 4 hours because, in theory, rapid-acting insulin has a duration of 3–4 hours. Yet different people metabolize insulin at different rates. Insulin pumps allow you to customize this setting. In pregnancy, you may find you need to shorten the insulin duration as a way to counteract pregnancy hormones and be more proactive in correcting higher blood glucose.

- **Extended Bolus—** This feature is unique to an insulin pump and allows for greater flexibility to be able to dose insulin based on the type of food. An extended bolus refers to an advanced way of delivering insulin so that it splits the bolus and gives part of it up front and the rest over an extended period. Most pumps have this feature, also known as dual-wave bolus. It is commonly used for high-fat foods; thus, the name "pizza bolus," since meals with a lot of fat can slow the absorption of carbs are raise blood glucose several hours later.

Continuous Glucose Monitors

CGMs have been a game changer in the diabetes world. Thanks to technology, we now have wearable devices that allow you to know your blood glucose level at all times without the need to repeatedly prick your finger. CGMs monitor the body's blood glucose in real time by sensing the glucose present in the tissue. They not only provide a blood glucose number, but can also capture the trend of change. The benefits of CGMs are many, but the main ones are improved A1C without an increase in low blood glucose and overall improved health of your baby. (Not to mention you will be able to save a few extra finger checks with the use of a sensor!)

In general, CGMs consist of a sensor, transmitter, and receiver. CGMs monitor blood glucose in real time by sensing the glucose present in the tissue. The sensor is inserted just under the skin and transmits blood glucose readings every 3–5 minutes to either a small handheld receiver or your phone. Most can be worn for up to 10 days. CGMs provide about 288 measurements of blood glucose per day![5] When used *in addition* to blood glucose testing before and after meals, CGMs can help improve A1C targets in diabetes and pregnancy.[4] Continuous glucose monitoring metrics should not be used as a substitute for self-monitoring of blood glucose to achieve optimal pre- and postprandial glycemic targets, however, they can decrease the frequency of tests.

Studies show that women with type 1 diabetes who use continuous glucose monitoring during pregnancy have improved neonatal outcomes. In other words, moms spent more time in target, had less high blood glucose, and their babies had better outcomes at delivery.[4] A study done in pregnant women with types 1 diabetes (the CONCEPTT study[6]) showed fewer large-for-gestational-age babies and less low blood glucose at birth (neonatal hypoglycemia) in mothers who wore a sensor compared to those who used finger sticks alone. Furthermore, women who wore a sensor spent 100 minutes a day longer in target compared to women who did not use a sensor.

Regardless of insulin delivery type, the use of a sensor improves blood glucose and lowers A1C.[7] Additionally, studies show that using CGMs can be cost-effective in the long run, especially if you are used to checking blood glucose multiple times a day.

However, not all women may be as open to trying a sensor. Possible barriers can include cost, fear of pain, or discomfort. The cost of one sensor out of pocket can range from $80 to $160, which adds up significantly over the course of a year. Fortunately, Medicare and private insurance providers now cover many sensors, though some will only cover a CGM if you are on multiple injections or have type 1 diabetes. (See Table 17.2 for an overview of the pros and cons of CGMs.)

For me, wearing a sensor throughout my pregnancy was very reassuring. I was able to see my blood glucose readings 24/7, which allowed me to understand my trends and make tweaks in my insulin dosage with my healthcare team. But the best part was that both my husband and I would get alerts when my blood glucose was falling in the middle of the night. In the end, there is no doubt that CGMs have revolutionized not only how we view diabetes, but also what we do to treat it. Based on the data available, wearing a real-time continuous monitor in pregnancy is recommended and can be beneficial.

TABLE 17.2 **Pros and Cons of CGMs**

Pros	Cons
• Data 24/7	• Cost
• Alerts for high and lows	• May not be covered by insurance
• Improved glycemic control	• May be overwhelming to have
• Less finger-stick checking	constant data on blood glucose
• Compatible with smartphone devices;	• May trigger fear of pain or discomfort
may allow you to share data with	• May result in adhesive reaction
other people	

Closed-Loop Insulin Delivery

Closed-loop systems, also referred to as an "artificial pancreas," or sensor-integrated pumps, are the newest diabetes technology. The hybrid closed-loop pump works by dosing basal/background insulin using a computer algorithm in response to real-time glucose measurements provided by the sensor. It essentially "closes the loop" by connecting the sensor and the pump. These systems still require carbohydrate counting and bolus delivery, but will automatically give insulin based on the sensor readings. The automation of insulin delivery can be a desirable feature in pregnant women where constant physiological changes require frequent insulin adjustments. Studies show that pregnant women with type 1 diabetes wearing a closed-loop insulin delivery system spent 15% more time in target at night and had less hypoglycemia compared to those wearing a traditional sensor and pump. In regard to labor and delivery, studies have shown a closed-loop pump performs well during labor, providing an 82% time in range, and 83% time in range postpartum. Despite these promising results, however, more studies need to be evaluated comparing closed-loop systems to traditional modalities in order to better understand outcomes.

Key Takeaways from This Chapter

✓ Diabetes technology has come a long way in the last 10 years. However, there is no *one* best technology tool for diabetes. The key is identifying the technology that fits and works for you.

✓ Insulin pumps provide continuous insulin delivery in pulse-like doses and allow for greater flexibility in insulin dosing

✓ If you are not using a pump but are interested, the best time to start is before pregnancy to give you enough time to troubleshoot and feel confident using it.

✓ Sensors have revolutionized diabetes management. Studies show that women with type 1 diabetes who use continuous glucose monitoring during pregnancy have improved neonatal outcomes.

✓ Closed-loop technologies are very promising and seem to be the future in diabetes care; however, as of now, there are limited studies focusing on pregnant women with diabetes.

REFERENCES

[1] Karges B, Schwandt A, Heidtmann B, et al. Association of insulin pump therapy vs insulin injection therapy with severe hypoglycemia, ketoacidosis, and glycemic control among children, adolescents, and young adults with type 1 diabetes. *JAMA* 2017;318(14):1358–1366

[2] Mukhopadhyay A, Farrell T, Fraser RB, Ola B. Continuous subcutaneous insulin infusion vs intensive conventional insulin therapy in pregnant diabetic women: a systematic review and metaanalysis of randomized, controlled trials. *Am J Obstet Gynecol* 2007;197(5):447–456

[3] Ranasinghe PD, Maruthur NM, Nicholson WK, et al. Comparative effectiveness of continuous subcutaneous insulin infusion using insulin analogs and multiple daily injections in pregnant women with diabetes mellitus: a systematic review and meta-analysis. *J Women's Health* 2015;24(3):237–249

[4] American Diabetes Association. 14. management of diabetes in pregnancy: *Standards of Medical Care in Diabetes–2019. Diabetes Care* 2019;42(Suppl. 1): S165–S172

[5] Draznin B (Ed.). *Diabetes Technology: Science and Practice.* Arlington, VA, American Diabetes Association, 2019

[6] CONCEPTT Collaborative Group. Continuous glucose monitoring in pregnant women with type 1 diabetes (CONCEPTT): a multicentre international randomised controlled trial. *Lancet* 2017;390(10110):2347–2359.

[7] Miller KM, Foster NC, Beck RW, et al. Current state of type 1 diabetes treatment in the U.S.: updated data from the T1D Exchange clinic registry. *Diabetes Care* 2015;38(6):971–978

CHAPTER 18

THE FIRST TRIMESTER— CONGRATULATIONS, BABY ON BOARD!

"My first thought when I found I was pregnant was 'Wait, What?' I knew it would happen, but I just didn't know it would happen this soon. I immediately called my endocrinologist. I knew I had to fine-tune my nutritional plan and work harder to get my blood glucose in tight control."

—Mariana Gomez, psychologist and project manager at Beyond Type 1, lives with type 1 diabetes and is a mom of a healthy boy.

Congratulations! You're having a baby! Excitement, fear, joy— you're likely experiencing all of those overwhelming emotions and more. So, let's take a deep breath: You got this! The journey begins now.

In this chapter, we will review step by step what is happening in your body and what to expect with your diabetes in the first 12 weeks of pregnancy. This first trimester is associated with lower blood glucose than usual, and many women may also experience hypoglycemia unawareness, not to mention morning sickness—all of which put you at risk of lows. As you read on, you'll find nutritional strategies as well as insulin/pump tips to consider to keep blood glucose in range. (For additional information, check out section 4, "Resources for All," where you'll find more about nausea, hypo-glycemia, and constipation.)

What to Expect in the First Trimester

- Feeling hormonal (extra progesterone is to blame).
- Possible morning sickness (like any other pregnancy).
- A 10%–20% decrease in insulin needs, since glucose crosses the placenta at a rate faster than average.
- The insulin phenomenon—you might start to produce insulin, which also causes lower blood glucose than usual.
- Potential hypoglycemia unawareness—reduced adrenal/sympathetic response, feeling tired, sluggish, and less likely to exercise.

During these first 12 weeks, your body is going through a lot of changes, particularly in the first 8 weeks. Even though your belly might not be showing yet, your body is preparing for what's ahead. By week 6, your baby's neural tube is closed, and your body is working hard to form your baby's lungs, heart, and brain. It's in these first 6–8 weeks after conception that you will make your first appointment to see your OB-GYN. During this first visit, expect to get an ultrasound to confirm the age of the baby. Additionally, you will get baseline labs like A1C, thyroid, and urine tests to check for kidney health. An echocardiogram might be recommended at this time if you have risk factors for heart disease, high blood pressure, or are older. If you haven't met with a registered dietitian or a diabetes educator, now is the time to do so. A registered dietitian will help you review carbohydrates, discuss essential nutrients in pregnancy, warn you about foods to avoid during pregnancy, and work with you to understand trends in blood glucose before and after meals. By the end of the first trimester and around week 12–16, you might be told to start low-dose aspirin as a preventative measure to lower the risk of high blood pressure in pregnancy, known as preeclampsia.

Nutritional Strategies in the First Trimester

For many women, the first trimester is the most challenging, as far as nutrition goes, due to nausea, vomiting, and possibly lower blood glucose. If you have not yet met with a registered dietitian or diabetes care specialist, use this time to relearn important nutrition concepts you might not have considered since diagnosis. You can refresh on carbohydrate counting and reading labels, and also fine-tune your diabetes skills. Below are other nutritional strategies to consider during this first trimester:

- Review carb counting. Every carbohydrate counts!
- Reread labels or invest in a food scale.
- If you are experiencing nausea/vomiting, aim for smaller but more frequent meals that are bland in taste, and choose cold foods instead of hot.
- Keep measuring cups handy, or even inside cereal boxes and oatmeal containers.
- Include nonstarchy veggies at all meals if possible.
- Focus on slow carbs and pair them with fats and/or protein.

The Insulin Phenomenon and Hypoglycemia Unawareness

You are more likely to experience hypoglycemia during the first trimester than any other time during your pregnancy. The difficulty for women with diabetes is that hypoglycemia during the first trimester is commonly associated with lower blood glucose propagated by morning sickness, an increase in insulin production, and a reduced ability to detect lows. In fact, severe hypoglycemia is three times more frequent in early pregnancy than before pregnancy, and is usually highest in weeks 8–16.[1]

Some women with type 1 diabetes start producing insulin during the first trimester of pregnancy.[2,3] It's somewhat of a medical mystery, but your formerly "defunct" pancreas all of a sudden starts producing insulin in this first trimester, which puts you at higher risk for hypoglycemia. For many women, hypoglycemia is more likely to occur at night. Consider decreasing long-acting insulin or reducing your basal rates at night. Make sure you keep track of your blood glucose and/or sensor data, and if you are noticing lower blood glucose, talk to your provider to change dosages accordingly.

Additionally, in these first weeks, you may notice that you are less likely to detect low blood glucose. This is referred to as hypoglycemia unawareness. The longer you live with diabetes and the tighter control you have, the harder it becomes to detect low blood glucose.

My Severe Hypoglycemia Scare

In the first 12 weeks of my pregnancy, I went to my hometown of El Paso, Texas, to visit my family. That weekend, we went to Ciudad Juarez, Mexico, for a Sunday lunch. I had fish, rice, and some veggies at one of my favorite restaurants—nothing out of the ordinary. I bolused early as I usually did, but I didn't finish all of my meal because I felt a little nauseous halfway through. I knew I had to eat something else to prevent me from going low, so I took a few sips of my sister's regular lemonade. Leaving the restaurant, I started to feel sick—so much so that we had to stop in the middle of the road because I needed to throw up. I looked at my sensor, and I was already at 60 mg/dL. Things were not looking good.

We were next to a supermarket, so my family got me some juice and Gatorade to bring my blood glucose up. I drank some and waited. Ten minutes later, I threw up again, and my blood glucose started to plummet. I began to panic; I was in the middle of a road in Mexico with no glucagon, unable to keep anything down, and my blood glucose was not going up. I started to explain to my family what to do if I were to pass out, when suddenly I had the idea to put honey in my mouth. I asked my husband to get me some. I placed it in my mouth, and sure enough my blood glucose slowly started to stabilize. Finally, we went back home, where I was able to get medication to stop the vomiting. Turns out, the next day, my family started feeling sick. It was a stomach virus that hit us all. Afterward, I always made sure to carry glucagon with me. I recommend carrying a fast-acting carbohydrate with you at all times, because you never know what could happen. Lessons learned: If you travel, always bring glucagon, train your family, and be extra prepared!

Before pregnancy, you might have been able to sense when you were going low. Sweating, irritability, hunger, faintness—you know the symptoms. However, during pregnancy, hypoglycemia unawareness is more prevalent. The reason is that the sympathetic response of hormones that raise blood glucose, like adrenaline and cortisol, is blunted. Usually, when your blood glucose is dropping, the body signals you by activating glucagon, growth hormones, and cortisol, among other hormones. In turn, this causes heart palpitations, sweating, and other symptoms. In pregnancy, this mechanism does not work as well, so by the time your blood glucose is down in the 50 mg/dL range, you're already confused because you never got the initial signals. This makes it an important time for your partner to become familiar with signs of low blood glucose as well as how to use glucagon.

Morning Sickness and Other Unpleasant Side Effects

Other unpleasant side effects like morning sickness, constipation, and heartburn are likely to appear at this time. But on the flip side, your hair becomes shiny and thick, and your skin takes on that pregnancy "glow" that people always comment on. You win some, you lose some! The increase in hormones (estrogen and progesterone) is to blame. A little Physiology 101: progesterone relaxes your muscles, which is why you experience heartburn and constipation. Keep in mind that if you are already experiencing morning sickness, you are at an even higher risk of experiencing low blood glucose. Below are some tips to help you avoid low blood glucose, but make sure to read the next section, "Resources for All," where we will go in-depth on all the side effects associated with pregnancy.

Quick Tips to Help Prevent Hypoglycemia
- Always carry a source of rapid-acting sugar, and make sure it's something that won't make you nauseous.

- Have glucagon available at all times.
- Carry starchy snacks like saltine crackers in your purse to help with nausea and prevent lows.
- If you are experiencing vomiting, consider taking insulin after your meal—once you're sure you've tolerated the meal and kept the carbohydrates in. Similarly, you could consider injecting half of the dose before the meal and the other half afterward.

Insulin Pump & CGM Strategies in the First Trimester

- Consider lowering your basal rates by 10%–20%, particularly at night. Hypoglycemia might be more prevalent at night.
- Increase your sensor's "low" setting to a higher number, and increase low blood glucose alarms to 80–90 mg/dL. That way, you are extra prepared when your blood glucose is reaching 90 mg/dL.

How to Stay Sane in the First Trimester

This first trimester can be a real awakening, because now it's real. Your blood glucose no longer affects just you, but also your baby. This added pressure to achieve "perfect blood glucose" can take a toll on your emotional and mental health. But repeat after me: *You don't need to have perfect blood glucose to have a healthy pregnancy.* In fact, there is no such thing as perfect blood glucose! Remember, many factors affect your blood glucose, especially during pregnancy, and not all of them are under your control (See Table 2.1, Factors That Affect Blood Glucose, on page 28.)

The important lesson is to adopt healthy coping skills and set realistic expectations during this stressful time. Take small steps and try to discover the source of your stress and where it's coming from. Once you identify the problem, it's easier to formulate a solution with the help of your diabetes team and loved ones. Make sure to reach out to friends and family or talk to your partner about how you are feeling. Take it one day at a time, and keep going!

My Husband's Advice to Other Partners

First, let me congratulate you: This will be an incredible adventure for you both. After going through this journey twice, I can tell you that the partner's role is vital every step of the way.

You have two goals: First, make sure she feels you support her unconditionally and help her make the process as enjoyable as possible. Easier said than done, I know. A regular pregnancy has challenges, and pregnancy with diabetes brings additional trials.

Let me share a few suggestions regarding the first goal:

- *Be involved. Attend as many doctor appointments as possible, educate yourself as much as you can about diabetes in pregnancy, and be ready to be her sounding board on how to approach challenges.*
- *Be supportive. Join her in the new daily routines such as afternoon walks to lower blood glucose or a new meal schedule.*
- *Be alert. With so many things going on, it's easy to lose track of key events and issues (sticking to the meal schedule, following her diet, more hypoglycemia than usual, etc.).*

The second goal is broader and more difficult: minimize stress and focus on what matters. There are so many factors that can introduce stress and ambiguity in diabetes. Your energy should focus on what is essential and necessary. I often found myself seeking to calm my wife and reassure her that things were going to be okay. We then focused on ways to improve things and not just worry about them. One factor to be aware of is the social pressure to comply with norms and customs imposed by family, friends, and even social media. Make sure these distractions don't become an unnecessary burden on you both.

Remember that this is a journey that must be tackled one challenge and day at a time. What feels like the hardest test today will be forgotten and replaced with another even more difficult challenge tomorrow (such as changing diapers during high turbulence in an airplane bathroom). Godspeed, and embrace the ride. You've got to be her rock!"

First Trimester Checklist

- Keep food and blood glucose logs.
- Meet with your OB-GYN to get prenatal labs, including A1C, 24-hour urine, and thyroid.
- Always keep a source of fast-acting carbohydrate with you

(in your car, purse, bag, etc.).

- Meet with a registered dietitian to review essential nutrients, carb counting, and foods to avoid.
- See an ophthalmologist for a dilated retinal exam.
- Meet with your endocrinologist and diabetes educator to review pregnancy goals, troubleshooting, and more.
- Expect to get lots and lots of ultrasounds. (At least you're able to see your baby more often!)
- If you don't yet have a sensor, consider the pros and cons.

Key Takeaways from This Chapter

✓ Check blood glucose more consistently due to hypoglycemia unawareness. If wearing a sensor, consider changing hypoglycemia settings to a higher value.

✓ Decrease basal insulin needs and insulin-to-carb ratios.

✓ Practice carb counting, reread labels, and remeasure food.

✓ Have a schedule for meals and try not to delay meals to avoid nausea.

✓ Keep fast-acting carbs at hand.

REFERENCES

[1] Nielsen LR, Pedersen-Bjergaard U, Thorsteinsson B, et al. Hypoglycemia in pregnant women with type 1 diabetes: predictors and role of metabolic control. *Diabetes Care* 2008;31(1):9–14

[2] Nielsen LR, Rehfeld JF, Pedersen-Bjergaard U, et al. Pregnancy-induced rise in serum C-peptide concentrations in women with type 1 diabetes. *Diabetes Care* 2009;32(6):1052–1057

[3] Ilic S, Jovanovic L, Wollitzer AO. Is the paradoxical first trimester drop in insulin requirement due to an increase in C-peptide concentration in pregnant Type I diabetic women? *Diabetologia* 2000;43(10):1329–1330

THE SECOND TRIMESTER—
BUMPY ROAD AHEAD

"I recall having a higher-than-normal blood glucose during my second trimester, and I was very nervous. At my next appointment, I shared my concern with my specialist. His reply: 'Your blood glucose was high for three hours, Ana. Not three days, not three weeks. When you saw it rising, you reacted appropriately and brought it down. You have not caused any harm to your baby.'"

—Ana Norton, diabetes advocate and founder & CEO of Diabetes Sisters, lives with type 1 diabetes and is a mom of a healthy boy.

Hello, baby bump! At last, you are now seeing your belly grow, making pregnancy all the more real. The second trimester, especially the first few weeks, is what I call the "honeymoon of trimesters." You're feeling more energized, and hopefully by now morning sickness has subsided. For the majority of women, morning sickness disappears by week 13 or 14. (If it hasn't, make sure to talk to your doctor to discuss ways to manage your nausea/vomiting.) You may also be feeling hungrier, and you're likely starting to add more weight, as expected. Every week, you will see your body change. Not to worry; a tiny human is growing inside of you.

For many women, the first trimester is the most challenging, due to nausea, vomiting, and possibly lower blood glucose. The second trimester is characterized by consistent trends in blood glucose with an increase in basal and bolus/food insulin requirements as the placenta hormones kick in. Up until now, your insulin dosages have been the same or are even lower than pre-pregnancy. In this second trimester, however, expect to see some changes in your insulin needs. Expect to have frequent insulin adjustments by the middle to end of this trimester. Bumpy road ahead!

In this chapter, we will review what to expect in weeks 13–28. We will highlight nutritional strategies to help with hunger and blood glucose spikes. At the end, we will evaluate insulin pump and continuous glucose monitoring tips to keep blood glucose in range.

What to Expect in the Second Trimester

- Less nausea/vomiting, feeling more energized.
- Increased hunger, might experience cravings.
- Ultrasounds about every 2–3 weeks.
- Around weeks 18–24, expect to see increases in insulin needs, especially in food/bolus insulin (the "diabetogenic stress" of pregnancy begins). Expect the biggest peak toward the end of the second trimester.
- Constant changes in basals, with a need to adjust every 2–3 weeks.
- More significant stress as you are dealing with frequent insulin changes.
- Gaining 1/2–1 lb per week on average (may be more or less depending on BMI and weight status before pregnancy).
- Mid-trimester glycemia will be the best predictor of your baby's size.

In this second trimester, you will see your doctor more frequently. The good news is that by week 20, you can know the sex of your baby. By week 24, expect to see your doctor every 2–4 weeks; after week 25, you might see your doctor every week. Tests at this time include a fetal anatomy test, where they will measure your baby's body parts, and a fetal echocardiogram, where you will go to a pediatric cardiologist and they will check that your baby's heart is doing okay. Sometimes, the extra glucose can accumulate in the form of plaque in your baby's arteries—another reason to keep blood glucose from becoming too elevated. See Table 19.1 for more information on prenatal visits.

Unlike the first trimester, when your insulin doses were pretty much the same or even lower, in this trimester you will start to see an increase in insulin demand. Don't worry: This is normal and expected in pregnancy. Pregnancy hormones kick in during the second

TABLE 19.1 Summary of Prenatal Visits

	When to see the OB-GYN	Tests to expect
First trimester	6–8 weeks after conception	Ultrasound Heart beat Due date
Second trimester: Week 20–24	Every 2–3 weeks	Gender reveal Echocardiogram Anatomy
Second trimester: After week 25	Every week	Non-Stress Test (NST) Biophysical Labs
Third trimester: Week 32–40	Twice weekly	Non-Stress test (NST) Biophysical labs

Source: Adapted from Ghirloni, S. Planning & Managing your Pregnancy. Joslin Diabetes Center.

trimester, which is when you will start noticing higher blood glucose and will require frequent adjustments in insulin doses. The pressure to keep tight blood glucose control 24/7 can leave you feeling isolated, vulnerable, and emotionally drained—not to mention that the surge of hormones is not helping. Be aware of your feelings and realize this is expected in a normal pregnancy. You just need to learn how to manage it. Now is a good time to find emotional support, whether it's keeping a journal, meditating, or simply talking to friends and family about how you're feeling. Realize you are not alone. Above all, be kind to yourself and focus on the big picture.

Nutritional Strategies

Welcome back, appetite! If you are feeling hungrier, it's with good reason: Your body now requires an additional 300 calories per day. The second trimester is the best time to get your routine set. Start exercising and be consistent with meals and snacks to keep you satisfied throughout the day. Three hundred calories is not that much food—it's an extra sandwich or a Greek yogurt topped with fruit and nuts. So the old phrase "eating for two" does not apply.

My golden rule for snacks is what I call the "FFP Rule": fat, fiber, and protein. Including snacks that have one of these three nutrients will help stabilize blood glucose and satisfy hunger. Fat, fiber, and protein all help you stay fuller longer. At this time, you may also want to make nonstarchy vegetables your best friends. Including plenty of lower-carbohydrate veggies at meals and snacks is a great way to curb hunger without impacting your blood glucose. (More information on snacks can be found in the next section, "Resources for All.")

And of course, a pregnancy would not be complete without the infamous cravings. It's not uncommon for pregnant women to have cravings, but in the case of women with diabetes, it can get a little tricky. I know what you are thinking: *"I have diabetes. I can't possibly eat my favorite foods!"* That certainly was not the case for me, nor does it need to be to sustain stable blood glucose. I had the opportunity to travel to Italy and I ate pizza and gelato in my second trimester, if that gives you hope. Being in the land of gelato and pasta seemed an impossible thing to negoatiate, but after talking to my healthcare team, we created a plan looked like this: lots of walking, earlier meals, great carb-counting skills, and early bolusing. With careful planning and lots of support, I was able to maintain amazing blood glucose. Having diabetes and being pregnant does not mean you can never enjoy your favorite foods. That said, it will require careful planning and evaluation. If you'd rather not go through the trouble of eating "problematic food," that's fine too. The point is that you may still be able to enjoy your favorite foods by changing the way it's prepared (e.g., less fat, lower carbs, or using natural fruit versus added sugars), changing the portion size, or eating it for lunch instead of breakfast (i.e., choosing a different time of day). With the help of a diabetes educator and registered dietitian, you will find you can still enjoy food during your pregnancy. And if you need inspiration for delicious treats that won't be detrimental to your diabetes, make sure to check out chapter 28, "Tasty Meal Plans."

Nutritional Strategies in the Second Trimester

1. Consider the importance of snacks to meet dietary needs.
2. Focus on FFP—fat, fiber, and protein—in all snacks.
3. Nonstarchy veggies with protein or fat will help you fill up.
4. Consider having a bigger lunch and lighter dinner (fewer carbs at night).
5. Acknowledge cravings rather than suppress them. Allow yourself to have something you enjoy—just make sure you eat it at the time it is easiest to manage blood glucose and have a plan in place.

Insulin Pump Tips to Help Keep Blood Glucose in Range

Up until now, your insulin doses might have been the same as, or even lower than, pre-pregnancy. In this trimester, however, expect to see changes in your insulin needs by week 18 or 19. By the end of the second trimester (around week 26), pregnancy hormones—in particular cortisol and human placental hormone—peak and will have the strongest effect on diabetes (also known as diabetogenic stress). As your placental hormones increase, your body will experience a greater need for insulin to keep up with your baby's demands. Injecting or bolusing before meals (20-30 minutes before) will take on even greater importance as blood glucose becomes a little more challenging to manage. At this time, you may also need to start increasing basals at night since pregnancy hormones are starting to kick in. Make sure you are keeping records of your blood glucose and food, as this data will help your medical team track patterns and make the necessary adjustments.

The second trimester is also crucial because your blood glucose control and weight gain during these weeks will predict the size of your baby. What this means is that if your blood glucose and weight remain steady, there is a better chance for your baby to have a healthy weight at delivery. On average, expect to gain about 1/2–1 lb every week after the first trimester (this may vary depending on pre-pregnancy BMI). Remember, the last trimester is mostly for growth, and your belly will expand. Every woman will gain weight at a different rate, though. Your doctor might recommend that you gain more weight if you started your pregnancy with a lower weight, or you might be told to gain less weight if your pre-pregnancy weight/BMI was higher. Just make sure your healthcare providers keep track if you are gaining appropriately. Below you will find other strategies to keep in mind as you progress into the second trimester of pregnancy.

Insulin Pump & CGM Strategies in the Second Trimester

- Bolus 20–30 minutes before meals.
- Adjust basals first, then carb ratios.
- Dual-wave bolus or split the meal to help postmeal blood glucose.
- Make sure you are keeping logs.
- You might need to increase night basals as your pregnancy hormones start kicking in, but everyone is different.
- Be mindful when treating hypoglycemia to avoid rebounds (might need 5–10 g of carbs versus 15 g).
- Consider changing the insulin duration (also known as "insulin on board") on your pump if you are experiencing higher blood glucose to facilitate quicker correction.

Staying Active

Being active will not only help you maintain a healthy weight; it will also decrease the risk of preeclampsia and C-section delivery, improve cardiovascular health, and help reduce those stubborn after-meal spikes. Think of exercise as another form of medication to lower blood glucose. Before pregnancy, you might have adjusted your insulin levels before or after activity, or even eaten a snack to prevent hypoglycemia. In pregnancy, however, you will notice this might not be the case. You probably will not need to decrease insulin or even have a snack (for fear of hypoglycemia), because you are probably not going to go low. Exercise will be a great tool to help manage blood glucose and make you more sensitive to insulin.

Going for a quick walk after meals can help reduce postmeal blood glucose, not to mention help boost your mood and relieve stress. Moreover, exercise helps you build the flexibility needed during labor, as well as the muscle tone that makes insulin work better. Finding ways to stay active in everyday life, even if it's just stretching or taking a short walk after meals, will make a difference. Check out chapter 12, "Exercise and Staying Active," to find out practical ways to fit 30 minutes of exercise in your daily routine.

Physical and Mental Benefits of Exercise

- Helps maintain weight
- Helps prepare you for labor and delivery (shorter labor)
- Lowers blood pressure
- Aids in relieving constipation
- Helps posture
- Improves mood
- Reduces anxiety
- Helps you sleep better

Key Takeaways from This Chapter

✓ Bolus 15–20 minutes before meals. The timing of insulin is equally or even more important than counting carbs.

✓ Be proactive in adjusting insulin dosages. If you notice a trend after 2 days, you might need an adjustment. Keep detailed logs and be in constant communication with your team. Don't wait weeks until contacting your healthcare team to make adjustments.

✓ Blood glucose might be more challenging to keep in target due to the increase in pregnancy hormones occurring during the second trimester. Recognize how you are feeling and find emotional support. You are not alone!

✓ When snacking, choose veggies using the FFP Rule, which suggests a small portion of protein, healthy fat, or slow carbs.

✓ Expect to get more tests in this trimester, including ultrasounds, fetal echocardiograms and anatomy tests, especially after week 24. You might need to see your doctor every 2–4 weeks.

THE THIRD TRIMESTER—
THE LAST *STRETCH*!

*"The last trimester can be really tough. My insulin
needs tripled; I was using an insulin-to-carb ratio of 1 unit
of insulin for every 2 grams of carbs! I had to be really
careful what I ate. It was hard in the moment, yes,
but oh so worth it! What kept me going was knowing
it was temporary and I'd get to enjoy all the carbs
I wanted as soon as she was born!"*

—Mary Ellen Phipps, registered dietitian and founder of Milk & Honey Nutrition,
lives with type 1 diabetes and is a mom of two healthy girls.

Only a few more weeks remain until showtime! By now,
you are feeling those baby kicks constantly and are thankful
for stretchy pregnancy pants. This last trimester is what I call
the "growth trimester." During these last weeks, your baby will gain
the majority of its weight. It's gone from the size of a peanut to the
size of a baby; that's a lot of change. And with this growth comes
insulin resistance, so expect to see major shifts in insulin needs.
Don't be surprised if, by this time, your insulin needs have tripled.
I went from an insulin-to-carb ratio of 1 unit for 9 g of carbs to 1 unit

for every 4 g. Significant increases in insulin needs are typical and expected, so make sure to be proactive and anticipate the increase in needs. Now is also the time to start familiarizing yourself with the labor protocol at your hospital. Ask about how they manage women with preexisting diabetes during labor and delivery.

In this chapter, we will review step by step what to expect in weeks 32–40. We will review the physiology of what is happening in this trimester and cover which tests should be performed at this time. Additionally, we will highlight nutritional strategies to help with insulin resistance and blood glucose spikes. Finally, we will discuss the importance of creating a birth plan and steps to get you ready to bring your baby home.

What to Expect in the Third Trimester
- High resistance to insulin: Insulin needs can triple.
- Insulin-to-carb ratios will change.
- The need to adjust insulin dosages every week.
- Greatest insulin resistance in the morning.
- Placental growth and contra-insulin hormones plateau at 36 weeks. After 36 weeks, expect similar trends in blood glucose and insulin needs.
- Progesterone slows down the digestion of food.
- Make sure to have your insulin prescription adjusted since the amount of insulin needed will increase.

Hello, Insulin Resistance!

This last trimester can be the hardest for women with preexisting diabetes because of the significant insulin resistance. Mornings can be especially challenging to your blood glucose as pregnancy hormones are at their peak. That said, you might need to reduce your carb intake in the morning to 15–30 g to keep blood glucose values in target range. Additionally, you may need to start taking insulin 30–45+ minutes before meals to prevent peaks. I know this can seem very frightening, but your healthcare team can support you in making the proper adjustments. Realize your body is going through drastic changes, which means your needs are changing drastically, too. Make sure you track foods and blood glucose and check in with your healthcare team often, as many adjustments will probably be made during this trimester.

By now, you are also probably getting fuller sooner because of your growing belly. Consider smaller meals to avoid heartburn. You can also consider splitting meals and taking the total insulin dose as a way to minimize the rises in blood glucose. For example, if you have an omelet with whole-wheat toast and yogurt in the morning, consider taking insulin to cover the whole meal, but just eating the omelet and toast, and then finishing the yogurt 1–2 hours later. This is mentioned in Diabetes Golden Rules in chapter 16, "Strategies to Avoid Spikes in Blood Glucose." Make sure you review these and more helpful strategies to avoid spikes in blood glucose.

Nutritional/Insulin Strategies in the Third Trimester
- Limit carbohydrates as needed, especially in the morning.
- Start with veggies first, then carbs.
- Split carbohydrate meals. Take a full dose of insulin, but split the meal into two.
- Consider a dual-wave bolus if you are eating a higher-fat/ -protein meal.
- Keep records of blood glucose, and expect to see steady increases in your insulin-to-carb ratios more so than basals.

At Your Doctor

After week 25, you will see your OB-GYN every week, but after week 32, get prepared to see them twice a week. You will probably alternate between your OB-GYN and your maternal-fetal medicine specialist (MFM). Moving forward, you will get a non-stress test at your doctor's visit. A non-stress test monitors your baby's movements and heartbeat. You will lie on your back, and a monitor will be placed on your belly to hear your baby's heartbeat. The test will last about 20 minutes, so bring a book or some type of entertainment. Additional tests will include a biophysical profile and amniotic fluid index, as well as routine urine tests.

As your due date approaches, you should become familiar with the delivery process. *Will you get to keep your pump and sensor? Who will be managing your diabetes? What is the treatment for low blood glucose if your baby were to experience it?* Don't be afraid to speak up if you feel strongly about a particular issue. Have an open discussion about the labor and delivery practices, but keep an open mind.

Creating a Birth Plan

If you suddenly feel the need to clean the baby's room, fix the crib, and wash all the baby clothes, you are probably going through the "nesting phase." This is common in the last trimester and serves an important role in getting you emotionally ready for bringing a tiny human home. Another way you can start getting psychologically prepared is through childbirth classes, as well as the creation of a birth plan. A birth plan is used to communicate your labor and delivery preferences to your healthcare team. In some cases, it can be a document; other times, it's simply a discussion. But the overall goal is to create a better experience and help inform your healthcare team of your personal choices.

Keep in mind, individual circumstances can arise that will deviate from this plan. Childbirth classes are a great way to learn about what to expect as well as basic and not-so-basic things about childcare, like learning to warm a bottle or clean a diaper. Breast-feeding classes can provide additional information on what to expect in those first days and can reduce the stress of not knowing.

Remember: Knowledge is power. I strongly encourage every new parent to attend childbirth classes mainly because you are already dealing with a lot of information for managing type 1 diabetes.

Birth Plan Checklist

General Questions/Considerations

- Who do you want alongside you?
- Will you want your baby to have skin-to-skin contact?
- In case your baby experiences low blood glucose at delivery, will you want them to give formula or breast milk?
- Will you use an epidural or other pain medications?
- Who will manage your diabetes during labor and delivery?
- How will the umbilical cord/placenta be handled? Special instructions?

What to Bring to the Hospital

- Comfortable clothes
- Type 1 supplies: medications and extra testing supplies (sensors, pumps, syringes, test strips, etc.)
- Nursing gear
- Nursing pillow or blanket
- Baby clothes with 2–3 changes
- Personal toiletries, including pads, as you might be bleeding
- Comfortable shoes, as your feet might be swollen
- Entertainment
- Going-home outfit
- Snacks
- Glucose tabs

Key Takeaways from This Chapter

✓ You may need to limit carbohydrates at breakfast since you will experience significant insulin resistance at this time.

✓ Eat your biggest meal at lunch/earlier in day instead of at dinner.

✓ It's easier to bring blood glucose up than to bring it down, so be mindful when treating lows.

✓ Walk after meals, as this can help prevent spikes after meals

✓ Timing of insulin may shift to 30–45 minutes before meals in order keep blood glucose in the 120-140 mg/dL range.

✓ Consider dual-wave bolusing to help extend coverage of insulin in a meal.

✓ Start planning for delivery by creating a birth plan.

CHAPTER 21

THE BIRTH—
IT'S GO TIME!

*"Don't assume you need to have a C-section.
The decision on a C-section should be
based on obstetrical need and not done solely
because you have type 1 diabetes."*

—Della Matheson, nurse and diabetes care specialist, lives with
type 1 diabetes and is a mom of three healthy kids.

R eady, set, go! After 9 months and a lot of love and hard work, the big day has arrived. You are probably wondering, *"Will I need to have a C-section?"* Being pregnant and having type 1 diabetes does not necessarily mean you will need to have a C-section. The time your baby arrives is based on many things, including the size of your baby, your medical team, the presence of complications, and individual preferences. Women with uncomplicated diabetes can safely deliver at full term (39–40 weeks); others may have a scheduled C-section at 38 weeks. Don't feel guilty or embarrassed if you need to have a C-section. (I had a C-section despite being in great control. More on this later.) What's important right now is not to lose sight of what matters most: having a healthy baby.

In this chapter, we will answer some of the most common questions: *"Will I need to have a C-section?" "Can I use my pump/sensor?" "What are the blood glucose targets at birth?"* We will review the different birth options as they relate to pregnancy with diabetes and discuss things to consider before arriving at the hospital.

What to Expect during Labor and Delivery

- Blood glucose target at delivery is 70–110 mg/dL.
- If your baby's weight is 4,500 g (>9 lb), consider a C-section.[1]
- Women with a well-controlled pregnancy and no complications can safely deliver at 39–40 weeks.
- Women with complications should consider earlier delivery at 36–38 weeks.
- If you are wearing a pump or CGM during labor, make sure you place it in an area that will not obstruct the doctors if they need to do a C-section.
- There will be a significant decrease in insulin needs immediately after giving birth.
- Insulin requirements return to the pre-pregnancy state once the baby is delivered. Make sure to account for this when setting basal programs.

Blood Glucose Targets and Delivery Options

One of my main concerns when I was pregnant with my first daughter was the actual birth. Having tight blood glucose control *during* labor is just as important as the past 9 months of hard work maintaining blood glucose in target. The recommended blood glucose target for labor is 70–110 mg/dL. Keeping tight control right up to delivery will also help your baby have normal blood glucose and avoid neonatal hypoglycemia. Babies of mothers with diabetes are at higher risk of having low blood glucose and may end up in the NICU in order to stabilize their blood glucose. Higher blood glucose at labor triggers your baby to start producing their own insulin, which could then result in neonatal hypoglycemia at the time of delivery.

In the past, women with preexisting diabetes were told they needed to deliver by a specific week. But thanks to modern advancements in diabetes monitoring, medications, and fetal tracking, there is less need for early delivery. According to the American College of Obstetricians and Gynecologists, women with well-controlled diabetes can safely deliver vaginally,[2] but this depends on several factors, including the presence of complications and baby size, among others.[1,3] After week 32, your OB-GYN may want to keep a closer eye on you by looking for any signs of preterm labor, monitoring your blood pressure (risk of preeclampsia), and tracking the size of your baby. A C-section might not be needed if your blood glucose remains in range and you show no signs of complication. The more in-target your numbers, the better you and your baby will be. If your baby is larger than expected, your doctor might want to induce labor or schedule a C-section ahead of time (usually around week 38) to avoid the risk of complications. Ultimately, what matters most is your health and the health of your baby.

Can I Use My Pump/CGM Sensor during Delivery?

Most hospitals have set protocols for the management of women with diabetes during pregnancy. If you are on multiple injections, you will likely be placed on intravenous (IV) insulin and IV dextrose (glucose drip) in case your numbers start to drop.[4] If you are wearing a pump, you may be allowed to continue to do so, but this decision will fall to the discretion of your doctor. Some medical teams have no problem letting you keep your pump, especially if you feel comfortable self-managing and can maintain target glucose numbers under 110 mg/dL.

Giving up control of your blood glucose can be very hard, especially if you are used to doing it yourself. I know for me personally, it was not easy, which is why I had an open discussion with my doctor. We created a plan for the big day in which I was allowed to keep both my pump and sensor, and the team (anesthesiologist, nurses, OB-GYN), including myself, kept close track of my sensor readings and pump the day of. Keep in mind, you are your own advocate. Don't be afraid to speak up if you feel strongly about keeping your pump/sensor. Have an open discussion about the labor and delivery practices, but keep an open mind. The decision to allow you to keep your pump/CGM really comes down to the discretion of the doctor and hospital.

Vaginal Birth

If you choose to have a vaginal delivery and have been cleared by your medical team, you will have a similar birth experience as women without diabetes, except your blood glucose will be monitored every hour. Expect your blood glucose to be very similar to the week before, since insulin needs will plateau after week 36. Placental growth stops after week 36, and the counterregulatory hormones plateau so that you won't see an increase in insulin needs beyond that point. If you are induced, oxytocin (Pitocin) will be given to begin contractions. You can choose to get an epidural early on, wait until later, or not get one at all; this is entirely your choice. If you are not using your pump, then two IVs will be placed: one with insulin and the other with dextrose in case your blood glucose starts to drop. Expect to see drastic drops in your insulin needs as soon as you give birth or just after.

What to Expect: Vaginal Delivery
- You may be induced at 39 weeks and given oxytocin (Pitocin) and other labor induction drugs to stimulate contractions and prepare your cervix.
- You will have a similar birth experience as women without diabetes. The main difference is your blood glucose will be checked more regularly.
- Take the usual bedtime dose of intermediate- or long-acting insulin.

- Do not take your morning dose of insulin and consider decreasing basals to avoid low blood glucose, depending on the time of delivery.
- Glucose will be checked hourly.
- If glucose is <60 mg/dL, dextrose IV will be given.
- You can choose to get an epidural.
- Expect blood glucose to remain the same as the week before— no major changes expected after week 36.
- Assign a person responsible for monitoring your sensor and managing your pump. Discuss this with the medical team.

C-section

If you are scheduled for a C-section, this will give you time to discuss the birth plan well in advance. Make sure to assign someone to monitor your blood glucose, or if you are keeping your pump, decide who will manage this during the surgery. Keep in mind that you need to be fasting for 12 hours before induction or a C-section, and no foods or drinks can be eaten. Therefore, the time of the surgery will matter. Ideally, early morning is best to decrease the time you will be without food. Morning basals will probably be reduced slightly (if you have a history of running lower in the morning) since you won't be eating anything, but again, this will depend on the time of the surgery.

During surgery, you will likely be placed on IVs, one with a dextrose drip and the other with an insulin drip (if not using the pump), to prevent your blood glucose from dropping or going too high. The surgery itself will last about 1 hour. Immediately after the surgery, your insulin needs will decrease significantly, so make sure to set the insulin rates in your pump close to how you had them set pre-pregnancy.

A C-section is considered major abdominal surgery, so make sure to take it easy afterward. The recovery will vary from woman to woman. Being active throughout your pregnancy will help you have a speedier recovery. After a C-section, you might experience the "shakes" or vomiting. (I did, and it was scary because I had no idea what it was.) It will be somewhat of a relief to have your blood glucose return to "normal" because you'll no longer have the increased insulin resistance you experienced in the third trimester. Nevertheless, you still want to keep your blood glucose as close to target as possible, as this will help the healing process. Take it easy for the next few days and enjoy time with your baby.

What to Expect: C-section

- A C-section is recommended depending on several factors, including the size of your baby, and kidney issues, among others.
- If scheduled, this will give you time to prepare in advance.
- Assign a person responsible for monitoring your sensor and managing your pump. Discuss this with the medical team.
- The time of the C-section is important since you will need to be fasting up until delivery. You need to fast for 12 hours before surgery.
- Take the usual bedtime dose of intermediate- or long-acting insulin.
- Do not take your morning dose of insulin and consider decreasing basals to avoid low blood glucose, depending on the time of delivery.

My Labor and Delivery Story

As I was reaching my third trimester, I was preparing myself for the physical aspects of having a natural birth. I was very active—walking, doing yoga—and my blood glucose never looked better. Things were looking up. I would dream of the moment I could hold my baby against my chest, and even imagined assisting my doctor in pulling my daughter out. That was what I thought would happen, but it didn't. At week 32, I was told I had placenta previa, which is when your baby's placenta partially or totally covers the cervix, making it very difficult for your baby to pass through. Placenta previa can cause severe bleeding during delivery. As a result, vaginal birth is contraindicated. At week 35, I got some good news: My placenta had moved, and I was cleared to have a vaginal delivery, expected around week 39. Things were looking good again! But at week 37, during my usual MFM visit, the doctor came back with bad news—my placenta had not moved the amount they wanted to clear me for a vaginal delivery. I was scheduled for a C-section the following week. Panic came over me. In my mind, I still had a good 2–3 weeks left, but now I was being told that I was to have a C-section the following Monday.

Of course, I was very disappointed, but as my doctor told me, "Marina, welcome to parenthood, where you are not in control of everything." This was, in fact, my first lesson in becoming a parent. My C-section was a success; my first daughter came into the world at 38 weeks and 2 days weighing 6 pounds, 13 ounces. Things don't always go as planned, and that's okay. Don't lose sight of what matters most!

Key Takeaways from This Chapter

✓ Women with uncomplicated diabetes can safely deliver at full term (39–40 weeks); others may have a scheduled C-section at 38 weeks. The most important goal is to have a healthy baby!

✓ Keeping tight control right up to delivery will also help your baby have normal blood glucose and avoid neonatal hypoglycemia. Aim to have blood glucose targets of 70–110 mg/dL during labor.

✓ You might be allowed to continue wearing your sensor and/or insulin pump during labor and delivery, but this decision will come down to your doctor and the hospital's protocol. Make sure you have a plan and discuss this with your doctor.

REFERENCES

[1] American College of Obstetricians and Gynecologists. ACOG practice bulletin no. 201: pregestational diabetes mellitus. *Obstet Gynecol* 2018;132(6): e228–e248

[2] American Diabetes Association. 14. Management of diabetes in pregnancy: *Standards of Medical Care in Diabetes—2019. Diabetes Care* 2019;42(Suppl. 1): S165–S172

[3] Spong CY, Mercer BM, D'alton M, et al. Timing of indicated late-preterm and early-term birth. *Obstet Gynecol.* 2011;118(2 Pt 1):323-333

[4] Stewart ZA, Yamamoto JM, Wilinska ME, et al. Adaptability of closed loop during labor, delivery, and postpartum: a secondary analysis of data from two randomized crossover trials in type 1 diabetes pregnancy. *Diabetes Technol Ther* 2018;20(7):501–505

THE FOURTH TRIMESTER—
BABY GOES HOME

*"Your emotional health and preparedness for what
comes next is as just as important as the 9 months before.
Make sure you always check your blood glucose before
breastfeeding because you are likely to have
lower blood glucose. Yes, your baby will be hungry
and cry (a lot), but making sure your blood glucose is
okay before feeding will be a priority!"*

—Mariana Gomez, psychologist and project manager at Beyond Type 1,
lives with type 1 diabetes and is a mom to a healthy boy.

Congratulations: You did it! Your baby is now home, and all those months of hard work and dedication paid off. Now, the work continues! In addition to taking care of this tiny baby, you still have your diabetes to manage. The "fourth trimester" refers to the period from the moment your baby is born up until three months of age. This period is known for its many changes as both you and your baby adjust to this new life. It can be very overwhelming, not to mention exhausting. *"Is my baby eating enough?"* *"Why is my baby crying?"* *"Am I doing this right?"* Being a first-time parent is filled with many doubts and a lot of anxiety. And this anxiety can cause your blood glucose to be out of whack. Remember, take a deep breath and take one day at a time. Every parent has gone through this before.

In this chapter, we will review the physical and emotional changes that you will encounter once your baby is born. These include hormonal changes, reduction in insulin needs, breastfeeding challenges, lack of sleep, anxiety, risk of postpartum depression, and family planning. Additionally, you will find helpful tips to help you breastfeed successfully.

What to Expect after the Baby is Born and Postdelivery Tips

- You will see a significant decrease in insulin needs. Expect to go back to pre-pregnancy doses or even lower if you are breastfeeding.
- If breastfeeding, your body requires an additional 400 calories per day.
- Have juice by your side and always carry fast-acting glucose with you.
- Consider liberalizing sensor glucose targets so the sensor is not continuously beeping. You need all the sleep you can get, so try to minimize additional sources of stress.
- Ensure you're eating nutrient-dense snacks throughout the day.
- Keep some high-fiber/high-protein granola bars on the bedside table.
- Sleep when the baby sleeps. Lack of sleep can affect you emotionally and make it harder to manage your diabetes.

Postdelivery Changes and Self-Care

One of the most significant changes you will notice is the sudden decrease in insulin needs. Don't be surprised if you need less insulin than you did pre-pregnancy, especially if you are breastfeeding. The extra calories burned while breastfeeding will be the equivalent of running 5 miles every day. If you are taking insulin, you will probably require half or one-third of the dose. For example, if you were taking 50 units of long-acting insulin during your last trimester, consider taking 20–25 units. Keep in mind that the insulin resistance you encountered in the last trimester instantly disappeared the moment you gave birth.

Emotional Sanity

Being a parent is hard work. Nobody taught you how to parent; you are learning as you go. It's not uncommon for new mothers to feel anxious and overwhelmed the first couple of months. For women with diabetes, managing your emotional sanity on top of your diabetes can be even more challenging. Furthermore, the influx of hormones post-delivery can also impact your mood. Many women experience "baby blues" a few weeks after birth or may develop a more serious case of postpartum depression. Symptoms include feeling overwhelmed, a sense of guilt, and difficulty sleeping. Make sure to talk to your doctor if you are feeling any of these symptoms and ask for help. You are not alone! Just remember to be aware of the symptoms, be kind to yourself, and don't expect perfection. If you need to loosen up your diabetes management, that might be okay. But make sure to talk to your doctor and healthcare team and see how they can help.

Breastfeeding

"Can I breastfeed if I have diabetes?" It's one of the most common questions for many women with diabetes. And the answer is an enthusiastic "Yes!" The American College of Obstetricians and Gynecologists HIGHLY recommends breastfeeding, as it's known to have many benefits for you and your baby. Breastfeeding will help you lose weight, improve insulin resistance, and boost your baby's immune system. Breast milk contains antibodies that protect your baby's immune system and reduce the risk of asthma, eczema, SIDS,[1] diabetes, celiac disease, and other allergic conditions.

What's more, you'll burn about 400 calories a day by breast-feeding. Yup, it's a lot of work! Be mindful that if you are breast-feeding, you are more prone to experience low blood glucose due to the extra demand for energy. Consider adjusting your insulin amounts in order to prevent hypoglycemia. You might also want to eat a carbohydrate snack before breastfeeding to keep your numbers from falling. See more ideas on breastfeeding snacks in section 4, "Resources for All."

Yet despite all of its known benefits, breastfeeding can be hard. For many women, it's not innate or natural in the first weeks. Plus, it can hurt, and it's emotionally and physically exhausting. But once you get the hang of it, it truly is a magical experience. For me, it wasn't easy initially, but thanks to the help of a lactation consultant, I knew what to expect and was able to do it successfully for almost a year. Successful breastfeeding will take practice, education, and determination. It's important to note that women with preexisting diabetes are at increased risk for lactation complications like mastitis, reduced milk production, and candida infections compared to women who don't have diabetes; the rates for exclusively breastfeeding in women with diabetes, primarily type 1 diabetes, are lower compared to mothers without diabetes.[2,3] Just know that if for whatever reason you decide not to breastfeed, that's okay, too. A growing and healthy baby is the most important thing. Below you will find some tips to prepare you and help you breastfeed with success.

Things to Consider when Breastfeeding

- Expect lower blood glucose, as your body is using more energy.
- Stay hydrated! Drink one glass of water at every feeding.
- Have carbohydrate-containing snacks before and/or after breastfeeding.
- Fuel up on wholesome, nutritious snacks, as your body is burning more calories.

Insulin Needs/Pump Settings during Breastfeeding

- Consider decreasing your daily basal.
- Decrease insulin-to-carb ratios to minimize lows.
- Consider a temporary basal before breastfeeding. If you are breastfeeding on demand, it might be easier to simply do a temporary basal for several hours.
- Keep in mind these needs can change. If you continue breastfeeding exclusively, your body might adapt to the insulin sensitivity, which will require you to increase your insulin doses.

Tips to Help You Breastfeed with Confidence and Success

- **Get informed.** Go to a breastfeeding class! This was the best thing we did. I got to know the myths, practiced positioning, and learned about latching. Check with your hospital or birthing place, as they usually offer them. Some may be free, while others can include a charge.
- **Don't wait to get help.** Find out if your hospital has a lactation consultant from day one.
- **Get to know hunger and fullness cues.** This will come with time and practice.
- **Make sure the baby is awake.** It might seem obvious, but this was a big lesson learned for me! This way, you make sure the baby gets a full feed. (I had to use a washcloth to wake up my oldest daughter.)
- **Trust!** This is the MOST important tip! You are not always in control. Trust your baby; trust in you. Trust you have enough breast milk. Trust your baby is eating what he or she needs.

Contraception and Family Planning

Part of your postpartum follow up should include seeing your OB-GYN to discuss a contraception plan. In case you are wondering, breastfeeding does not qualify as a safe contraception method. You can still get pregnant if you are breastfeeding! Planning pregnancy is critical in women with preexisting diabetes due to the need for tight blood glucose management before pregnancy to prevent congenital and birth malformations. After reading this section, you realize that pre-conception planning as well as tight diabetes management before conception are critical factors in reducing the risk of birth defects. Women with diabetes have the same contraception options and recommendations as those without diabetes. The biggest barrier for effective preconception planning is actually unplanned pregnancies. Because most pregnancies are unplanned, it's so important for women with diabetes to have family planning options reviewed to make sure effective contraception is implemented.

Key Takeaways from This Chapter

✓ Your emotional health and well-being once your baby comes home is a priority.

✓ Expect significant decreases in your insulin needs, especially if you are breastfeeding.

✓ Taking care of a tiny human on top of trying to manage your diabetes is overwhelming. Many women experience "baby blues" a few weeks after birth, or may develop a more severe case of postpartum depression. Make sure to talk to your doctor if you are feeling down and realize you are not alone.

✓ Breastfeeding will help you lose weight, improve insulin resistance, and boost your baby's immune system.

✓ Planning pregnancy is critical in women with preexisting diabetes due to the need for tight blood glucose management before pregnancy to prevent congenital and birth malformations.

REFERENCES

[1] Hauck FR, Thomson JM, Tanabe KO, et al. Breastfeeding and reduced risk of sudden infant death syndrome: a meta-analysis. *Pediatrics* 2011;128(1): 103–110

[2] Leahy, K. Postpartum Care, Lactation and Contraception in Diabetes. On the Cutting Edge. *Diabetes Care and Education* 2016;Vol 37(4):41–43

[3] Sparud-Lundin C, Wennergren M, Elfvin A, Berg M. Breastfeeding in women with type 1 diabetes: exploration of predictive factors. *Diabetes Care* 2011;34(2):296–301

Resources
for All

SECTION 4
Resources for All

WE'RE ALL IN THIS TOGETHER

This is a must-read section for all! After reading prior sections, you've realized that having a healthy and happy pregnancy is possible. You now have the knowledge and know-how to keep blood glucose in target without sacrificing the foods you love or your sanity. Hopefully, by now you feel empowered and confident to continue your pregnancy journey, whether you live with diabetes and are just starting to consider pregnancy or have been diagnosed with gestational diabetes. This section addresses topics for *all* pregnant women, regardless of the type of diabetes. At the end of the day, all pregnant women have one common goal: having a healthy baby.

The following chapters will help you understand common concerns that accompany pregnancy and will provide practical solutions on how best to manage them. We will cover things like morning sickness, essential nutrients during pregnancy, managing constipation, understanding nutrition labels, and debunk common myths in the Q&A chapter. Last, but not least, you will find ideas on hearty snacks, meal plans, and tasty recipes to try. So let's get started!

chapter 24

KEY NUTRITION PILLARS FOR <u>ALL</u> PREGNANT WOMEN

Pregnancy is a unique time in a woman's life where the body goes through a lot of physical changes. Proper nutrition plays an essential role in making sure both you and your baby are healthy. In these 9 months, your body will require certain nutrients to make sure your baby grows appropriately. As you've probably figured out by now, there is no "pregnancy diet" or "eating for two." Instead, the same healthy and balanced eating habits that worked pre-pregnancy continue to apply. However, there are some essential vitamins and nutrients that play a unique role during pregnancy, so you'll want to make sure to include them in your daily eating routine.

You might be surprised to know that the nutrient requirements for pregnant women with diabetes are the same as those for pregnant women without diabetes. Nevertheless, you might still have questions about whether you can include certain foods in your diet. *"Can I have fish?" "Is it ok if I drink coffee?" "Are non-nutritive sweeteners safe for my baby?"* In this chapter, we will cover common nutritional concerns during pregnancy and review the essential nutrients you should focus on before and during these 9 months. So, let's dive right in!

Folic Acid

Consider this mineral a superstar when it comes to your baby's development. Folate is naturally found in dark leafy vegetables and beans. Folic acid is the synthetic version found in enriched cereals and grains and is also included in your prenatal vitamin. Both folate and folic acid are responsible for the production of red blood cells, which are vital for your baby's spinal cord development. Inadequate folate and folic acid, especially in the first trimester, increases the risk of neural tube defects (spina bifida), low birth weight, and preterm birth, which is why folic acid supplementation is so necessary before pregnancy.

If you are considering pregnancy, one of the first things you should do is start taking a prenatal vitamin at least 2–3 months before conception. Studies have shown that consuming 400 mg of folic acid before and during pregnancy can reduce 50% or more of neural tube defects.[1] During pregnancy, folate needs increase to 600 mg, so make sure in addition to your supplement, you include folate-rich foods in your diet (Table 24.1).

TABLE 24.1 **Folate Needs at Various Stages**

	Folate (mg/day)
Nonpregnant	400
Pregnant	600
Nursing	500

Foods Rich in Folate

- Asparagus
- Beans/lentils
- Broccoli
- Cooked spinach
- Fortified cereal
- Fortified orange juice
- Strawberries

Protein

Proteins are the building blocks of our DNA. They are found in our cells, hormones, and enzymes. So, it comes as no surprise that protein needs increase during pregnancy; after all, you're making another human being. The recommended dietary allowance (RDA) for protein is based on your weight. On average, pregnant women need 71 g protein (or 1.1 g/kg of body weight). If you are having twins, protein needs go up even more: you need an additional 50 g protein per day. Protein can be found in foods such as eggs, fish, beef, and turkey, as well as in nonanimal, plant-based sources like beans, nuts, tofu, and quinoa, among others. Protein will have a minimal effect on your blood glucose;[2,3] however, in some women with type 1 and type 2 diabetes, consuming large amounts may impact blood glucose values, so keep an eye on this. Some plant-based proteins also contain carbohydrate, so be mindful and make sure to count them accordingly.

Foods Rich in Protein

- Beans*
- Cheese
- Chicken
- Eggs
- Fish
- Nuts
- Peanut butter

- Pork
- Quinoa*
- Soy milk and some plant-based milk alternatives*
- Tofu
- Yogurt*

(*contains carbs)

Calcium

Calcium is a critical mineral that is responsible for building your baby's bones, teeth, and nails. At the same time, calcium intake protects you from bone loss. As your baby continues to grow in the second and third trimester, the need for calcium goes up. The recommendation for pregnant and breastfeeding moms is to consume 1,000 mg of calcium a day. Interestingly, during pregnancy, your body senses the baby's increased need and is more efficient in absorbing calcium from food. The wonders of mother nature! Your baby will always get the calcium he/she needs from you, so if you don't consume enough calcium, this puts you at an increased risk for osteoporosis in the long run. Most prenatal vitamins have about 150 mg calcium, so make sure you take a prenatal supplement with calcium in addition to including foods naturally high in calcium.

Foods Rich in Calcium
- Almonds
- Broccoli
- Fortified plant-based milk, such as soy milk

- Milk
- Salmon, canned
- Sardines
- Tofu
- Yogurt

Vitamin D

Vitamin D goes hand in hand with calcium since it's responsible for keeping adequate calcium stores. If you're low in one, you might be deficient in the other. More important, people with diabetes tend to be lacking in vitamin D. There is an interesting connection between vitamin D levels, obesity, and autoimmunity. Low levels of vitamin D are commonly seen in newly diagnosed kids with type 1 diabetes.[4] At the same time, new evidence links obesity with low levels of vitamin D.[5] Vitamin D may have important roles in immunity that we don't yet fully understand. The RDA for vitamin D during pregnancy is 600 IU/day. Sunlight triggers vitamin D production, but many people living in sunny places are still deficient, so don't rely solely on sunshine. Additionally, having darker skin puts you at higher risk for low levels because your body produces more melanin, which blocks the production of vitamin D.

Foods Rich in Vitamin D
- Eggs
- Fortified cereal
- Fortified plant-based milk, such as soy milk
- Milk
- Mushrooms
- Salmon
- Yogurt

Omega-3/DHA

Docosahexaenoic acid (DHA) is a type of omega-3. It is critical in your baby's brain development during pregnancy, nursing, and even in the first years of life. Because the body can't produce DHA, it's essential we consume it in our diet. The RDA in pregnancy is 300 mg/day. Unfortunately, the majority of Americans don't get enough DHA.[6] According to the NHANES survey, most women only consume about 60 mg/day.[7] DHA is naturally found in many types of seafood, like sardines, salmon, and tuna. Recently, it's been added to milk, eggs, and yogurt products, so you might benefit from choosing those fortified products as well.

Foods Rich in DHA
- Flaxseeds
- Salmon
- Chia
- Walnuts
- Sardines
- Tuna
- DHA-fortified foods (milk, eggs, yogurt)
- Seaweed
- Trout

DID YOU KNOW?

Americans have the lowest intake of DHA in any developed country in the world. Make sure your prenatal supplement includes DHA and that you are evaluating your food accordingly. Six ounces of salmon provides around 1,200 mg of DHA—enough to meet your daily needs.

Choline

Choline is an essential nutrient that also plays a role in preventing neural tube defects. It's needed for cell metabolism, a healthy nervous system, and brain functioning. You need 450 mg in pregnancy and 550 mg during nursing.

Foods Rich in Choline
- Eggs
- Cod
- Beef
- Chickpeas
- Chicken
- Wheat germ

Iron

Iron is needed to make red blood cells and transport oxygen throughout the body. Iron is one of those minerals that is important during pregnancy and even more so during the first year of your baby's life. Iron requirements during pregnancy are notably higher than those of non-pregnancy: 27 mg/day versus 18 mg/day, respectively (Table 24.2). Extra iron is needed to keep up with your baby's red blood cell production. About 50% of pregnant women don't get enough iron. Your doctor will probably check iron levels during the first and last

TABLE 24.2 Iron Needs at Various Stages

	Iron (mg/day)
Nonpregnant	18
Pregnant	27
Nursing	9

trimesters to make sure you are not deficient. Most prenatal supplements include about 27 mg, but you still want to include foods high in iron in your diet. If you are vegetarian, vegan, or have any allergies, you could be at a higher risk of developing anemia.

> **TIP:** *Pair a plant-based source of protein (lentils, chickpeas, beans) with a food high in vitamin C (oranges, strawberries, broccoli, red peppers) to help increase iron absorption.*

Foods Rich in Iron

- Chicken
- Lentils
- Sweet potatoes
- Fortified cereal
- Oatmeal
- Soybeans
- Spinach
- Beef
- Lamb

Sodium

The recommended sodium amount for pregnant women is the same as for nonpregnant women: 2,300 mg/day. Keep in mind that if you are overweight or suffer from high blood pressure, sodium will be something to keep a close eye on. We know excess sodium intake is linked with high blood pressure. Being overweight and having diabetes in pregnancy increase your risk of developing preeclampsia, so it will be important to keep track of your sodium consumption to help manage your blood pressure. Most of the sodium we consume is in the form of processed foods, less so than the actual table salt you use to cook.

Strategies to Help Keep Sodium Levels in Check
- Try to buy fresh products when possible.
- If buying canned products, look for "low sodium" on the label.
- If buying frozen, look for options without added sauces.

Caffeine

Caffeine is a stimulant, and too much caffeine in pregnancy is associated with low birth weight and spontaneous abortion,[8] which is why it should be consumed in moderation. You might have heard that if you are pregnant, you need to eliminate coffee. But according to the 2015–2020 Dietary Guidelines, the suggested limit is under 300 mg/day. Depending on the type of coffee you drink, this is about 1 cup of American coffee or 1 1/2 shots of espresso. Not bad, huh? Although coffee can be a primary source of caffeine, other drinks like tea, soft drinks, and energy drinks, as well as some candies, can include caffeine too (Table 24.3).

DID YOU KNOW? A shot of espresso will have less caffeine than a regular cup of American brewed coffee. One ounce of espresso contains around 65 mg caffeine; 1 cup of American brewed coffee contains 165 mg of caffeine.

Nonnutritive Sweeteners

If you had diabetes prior to pregnancy, you are probably already familiar with nonnutritive sweeteners. They're used in place of sugar or honey to sweeten your coffee or yogurt. But what about during pregnancy? Are they safe for your baby?[9] Nonnutritive sweeteners are generally recognized as safe (GRAS) to use in moderation during pregnancy by the FDA. These include aspartame (Equal), stevia, sucralose (Splenda), saccharin (Sweet'N Low), and neotame.[10]

TABLE 24.3 Caffeine Intake in Common Drinks

	Size	Caffeine intake (mg)
Regular American brewed coffee	8 oz	95–165
Espresso shot	1 oz	47–64
Cappuccino	16 oz	150
Decaf Americano	8 oz	0
Decaf Espresso	1oz	0–15
Instant coffee	8 oz	63
Latte	8 oz	63–126
Green tea	8 oz	25–30
Black tea	8 oz	25–48
Regular soda	16 oz	25–75
K-Cup (most varieties)	1 K cup	75–150

Source: Adapted from Mayo Clinic. Caffeine content for coffee, tea, soda and more [Internet], c2020. Mayo Foundation for Medical Education and Research. Available from https://www.mayoclinic.org/healthy-lifestyle/nutrition-and-healthy-eating/in-depth/caffeine/art-20049372; and McCusker RR, Fuehrlein B, Goldberger BA, Gold MS, Cone EJ. Caffeine content of decaffeinated coffee. J Anal Toxicol. 2006;30(8):611-613.

Sugar Alcohols

Sugar alcohols are sweeteners commonly used in "low-calorie" or "sugar-free" products to enhance the taste and texture without the added sugar or carbohydrate. Similar to artificial sweeteners, they are safe to use in pregnancy. Sugar alcohols are a source of carbohydrate but are not fully absorbed by the gastrointestinal system. Only about half of the amount will impact your blood glucose. Consuming too much sugar alcohols can cause digestive problems like cramping, bloating, or diarrhea, so be wary.

Examples of Sugar Alcohols

- Erythritol
- Isomalt
- Maltitol
- Sorbitol
- Xylitol

> **TIP:** *Many common sugar alcohols will end in "ol" (e.g., sorbitol, maltitol), so look for ingredients ending in "ol" when trying to determine if a food contains sugar alcohols.*

Fish Consumption/Mercury

You might have heard you need to avoid *all* fish in pregnancy. Not true. Fish and seafood provide vital nutrients like protein, zinc, and omega-3, which are beneficial for your baby's brain development. Consistent evidence shows that eating a wide variety of seafood during pregnancy is associated with improved neurocognitive development in children compared to not eating seafood at all. Think of fish as a source of brain food for your baby.

A significant reason fish and seafood are controversial is because of the high mercury levels present in certain fish. Mercury is a metal commonly found in bigger predatory fish like shark, mackerel, bigeye tuna, and swordfish. Too much mercury in your system can be harmful to your baby's lungs, heart, and brain development. Because of this, there are certain fish you will need to avoid during pregnancy.

However, the FDA recommends a pregnant woman eat 8–12 oz of low-mercury fish like salmon, shrimp, tilapia, sole and pollock per week, which comes down to 2–3 servings per week to get enough omega-3/DHA. We know that the majority of pregnant women don't meet the recommended daily DHA amounts. Foods like salmon and sardines are some of my top recommendations for pregnant women in particular. Interestingly, one study found that even when women consumed higher amounts of fish (>12 oz/week), no adverse effects were reported,[11] which is always reassuring. Nevertheless, it's important to be mindful of mercury in fish, but there's no reason to altogether avoid low-mercury fish and seafood while pregnant (Table 24.4). Fish might also have a bad reputation due to the risk of foodborne illnesses if not cooked properly. If you are eating fish, remember to avoid any raw fish like sushi and tartare, which pose a high risk for food poisoning or contamination.

TABLE 24.4 Seafood to Eat or Avoid based on Mercury Levels

Low-mercury seafood (Eat)	Medium-mercury seafood (Eat in moderation: 6 servings or less/month)	High-mercury seafood (Limit: 3 servings or less per month)	Highest-mercury seafood (AVOID all)
Tilapia	Lobster	Bluefish	Marlin
Salmon	Mahi-mahi	Grouper	Shark
Pollock	Halibut	Tuna (canned albacore)	Ahi tuna (big eye)
Scallop	Tuna (canned non-albacore in water)	Tuna (yellowfin)	Swordfish
Shrimp	Snapper	Mackerel (Spanish/Gulf)	King mackerel
Sardine	Cod (Alaskan)	Sea Bass (Chilean)	Tilefish
Trout (freshwater)	Bass		
Sole			
Squid			

REFERENCES

[1] Committee on Genetics. Folic Acid for the Prevention of Neural Tube Defects. *Pediatrics* August 1999;104(2):325-327

[2] Institute of Medicine. *Dietary Reference Intakes for Energy, Carbohydrate, Fiber, Fat, Fatty Acids, Cholesterol, Protein, and Amino Acids*. Washington, DC, The National Academies Press, 2005

[3] Institute of Medicine, Food and Nutrition Board. *Dietary Reference Intakes: The Essential Guide to Nutrient Requirements*. Washington, DC, The National Academies Press, 2006

[4] Raab J, Giannopoulou EZ, Schneider S, et al. Prevalence of vitamin D deficiency in pre-type 1 diabetes and its association with disease progression. *Diabetologia* 2014;57(5):902-908

[5] Walsh JS, Bowles S, Evans AL. Vitamin D in obesity. *Curr Opin Endocrinol Diabetes Obes* 2017;24(6):389-394

[6] American Pregnancy Association. Omega 3 fatty acids: faqs [Internet]. Available from https://americanpregnancy.org/pregnancy-health/omega-3-fatty-acids-faqs/

[7] Thompson M, Hein N, Hanson C, et al. Omega-3 fatty acid intake by age, gender, and pregnancy status in the United States: national health and nutrition examination survey 2003–2014. *Nutrients* 2019;11(1):pii:E177

[8] Higdon JV, Frei B. Coffee and health: a review of recent human research. *Crit Rev Food Sci Nutr* 2006;46(2):101–123

[9] American Diabetes Association. 14. Management of diabetes in pregnancy: *Standards of Medical Care in Diabetes—2019. Diabetes Care* 2019;42(Suppl. 1): S165–S172

[10] Kaiser L, Allen LH; American Dietetic Association. Position of the American Dietetic Association: nutrition and lifestyle for a healthy pregnancy outcome. *J Am Diet Assoc* 2008;108(3):553–561

[11] Hibbeln JR, Spiller P, Brenna JT, et al. Relationships between seafood consumption during pregnancy and childhood and neurocognitive development: two systematic reviews. *Prostaglandins, Leukotrienes & Essential Fatty Acids* 2019;151:14–36.

MANAGING SIDE EFFECTS OF PREGNANCY—THE GOOD, THE BAD, AND THE UGLY

B eing pregnant is a beautiful thing, but it can often be accompanied by unpleasant side effects like nausea, constipation, and heartburn. About 50%–80% of all pregnant women experience morning sickness, characterized by nausea and vomiting. For the pregnant woman without diabetes, these side effects are just annoyances; but for the woman with diabetes, they involve more planning and can be challenging to manage.

In this chapter, we will discuss the not-so-pretty side of pregnancy that includes nausea, vomiting, constipation, and hypoglycemia, as well as helpful strategies on how to manage them. We will highlight issues relevant specifically to the woman with diabetes—hypoglycemia, treatment when vomiting, ketoacidosis—and we will discuss how they can best be treated.

Managing Nausea/Morning Sickness

Nausea and vomiting tend to occur in the early part of pregnancy and may subside by the second trimester. Although the exact cause of nausea during pregnancy is not really known, it's probably caused by the surge of hormones, making you more sensitive to smells and tastes. Morning sickness can be a tricky issue for women with diabetes. The biggest risk is the potential for dehydration and hypoglycemia, especially if you are taking insulin. Both hypoglycemia and vomiting are something to be taken seriously because they can quickly lead to ketones in the body, or diabetic ketoacidosis. If you are taking insulin and are unable to keep food down, you are at an even greater risk for severe low blood glucose. In these cases, you might need to take insulin after meals or split the dose. Make sure to carry glucagon with you at all times.

Morning sickness treatment and management is very individualized. The types of food that trigger it are totally different for each woman. Furthermore, the degree of nausea and/or vomiting varies greatly from woman to woman. Note that extreme vomiting, also known as hyperemesis, will require a different type of management, which can even include medication or hospitalization. The main point is to listen to your body and avoid foods that don't seem appetizing. Although there are some practices that can help nausea subside, the only real treatment is time. Below you will find helpful tips to alleviate and minimize the discomfort of nausea and vomiting.

Tips to Alleviate Nausea

- **Have small but frequent meals.** Nausea tends to be triggered when the stomach is empty, which is why having smaller meals more frequently will be better than large meals. Avoid large meals as they will only worsen nausea. Make sure to include a protein, fat, and slow carbs at meals to keep your blood glucose stable.

- **Have a snack before bed.** Similar to the point above, eating a snack before bed can help alleviate morning nausea. Make sure to include a protein or healthy fat like peanut butter or avocado to keep your stomach full for longer periods.
- **Ginger is your new best friend.** Ginger is one of the only nutritional interventions that has been shown to clinically reduce nausea. Options include ginger tea, ginger capsules, and ginger candy.
- **Take your prenatal vitamins at bedtime, not in the morning.** Some prenatal vitamins can exacerbate nausea. Consider changing them to a time when you are least nauseated, or take them once you have some food in the stomach. Ask your doctor about switching the type of vitamin to see if this can help.
- **Limit the caffeine and spice.** Strong flavors and odors can trigger nausea, so it's best to avoid spicy food. Caffeine is also shown to aggravate nausea.
- **Keep simple, starchy carbs close to you.** Think saltine crackers, cereal Os, toast, and rice cakes. Have some type of low-fat cracker in your purse or by your bedside in case you start feeling nauseous.
- **Stay hydrated.** Hydration is one of the most important things to maintain throughout your pregnancy, especially if you are experiencing morning sickness. Throughout the day, make sure to sip on fluids such as water or decaffeinated beverages, or munch on ice chips. If you are vomiting, you will also need to keep your electrolytes in balance, so sipping on sports drinks or broths, or even eating popsicles, will help you stay balanced.

Tips for Managing Vomiting

- **Decrease rapid-acting insulin before meals.** Consider read-justing your dosages if you are having constant episodes of nausea/vomiting and have a hard time keeping food down. Make sure you talk to your doctor right away.

- **Split insulin doses.** Consider taking half of the insulin at the start of the meal, and the other half at the end.
- **Ask about medication.** If you are experiencing severe and persistent vomiting, your doctor may prescribe medications to help manage this.
- **Consider glucagon.** In severe cases of low blood glucose where you are unable to keep any food down and blood glucose is not going up, you may need to consider taking a small dose of glucagon.

Constipation

Constipation is fairly common in pregnancy. This is partly due to the hormone progesterone, which slows the movement of food through your gastrointestinal system. Also, your prenatal vitamin may be to blame. Large doses of iron supplementation—like those in your prenatal—can also cause constipation. Also, you may be feeling more sluggish, and your physical activity could be limited, thereby increasing the odds of being constipated.

The best way to manage constipation is through the "MWF" rule: movement, water, and fiber:

- **Movement—**Being active will not only help your mood and help you avoid excessive weight gain, but exercise also gets your intestines moving. It's as simple as that! When you move, the extra blood flow will help move the backup in the stomach.
- **Water—**Dehydration is linked to premature labor and even preeclampsia, which is why being properly hydrated is so important during pregnancy. Make sure you are drinking at least 10 cups of fluid a day. This includes fluid from decaffeinated drinks, milk, tea, and even fruit and water-filled veggies.
- **Fiber—**Fiber will help move the food along through your stomach. Not only will it help you "unclog" your stomach, but it also

plays a key role in delaying the rise of glucose spikes. So, yay for fiber! Fiber also absorbs the fluid in your system, which is why you need to make sure you're drinking plenty of fluids. The recommended fiber intake is 28 g/day, yet the majority of adults only consume about half of this. Fruits and veggies are a natural source of fiber, or you may also need to add a fiber supplement if natural foods are not enough. Choose a psyllium fiber supplement. Look under dietary fiber when reading the nutrition label and aim for at least 2–3 g of fiber per portion! (For more on how to read a nutrition label, see chapter 26.)

Foods Rich in Fiber
- Avocado
- Beans
- Chia
- Lentils
- Oatmeal
- Whole-grain cereal

Heartburn

Heartburn is more common in pregnancy due to the hormone progesterone, which causes your muscles to relax. The burning sensation is caused when gastric acid from the stomach is pushed towards your esophagus. You are more likely to experience heartburn in the first trimester and the last trimester, where your expanding belly will put pressure on your stomach.

Tips to Alleviate Heartburn
- Sleep with your head and upper body elevated.
- Eat small, frequent meals.
- Avoid spicy, greasy, or fatty food, as well as caffeine.
- Wait 1 hour after eating before you lie down.

TABLE 25.1 Best Foods or Drinks to Treat Low Blood Glucose with 15 g of Carbs

Food	Carbohydrate (g)
3–4 glucose tabs	15
4–5 pieces of hard candy	15
4 oz juice	15
1 tablespoon honey	15

Hypoglycemia

Hypoglycemia is much more common in the first trimester of pregnancy in type 1 and type 2 diabetes, however if you are taking medication you are at higher risk of experiencing low blood glucose. In the event that you have a low blood glucose, make sure to follow the 15–15 rule for treating hypoglycemia: take 15 g of fast-acting carbohydrate (Table 2.4), and wait 15 minutes before testing again. Glucose tabs and honey are gentler on the stomach. Use these instead of juices if you are experiencing morning sickness. For more examples of foods/drinks to treat hypoglycemia, see Table 25.1.

Diabetic Ketoacidosis

Diabetic ketoacidosis (DKA) is a potentially life-threatening condition that occurs when there is a lack of insulin and the body is forced to break down fat for fuel. The by-product of this process is known as ketones. Having moderate or large amounts of ketones in the body makes the blood become acidic, which then could lead to respiratory distress or coma. DKA is usually the first sign of diagnosis for people with type 1 diabetes. During pregnancy, ketones can develop faster, which is why your doctor may want you to check them in the morning or any time your blood glucose reaches 250 mg/dL. DKA during pregnancy poses a significant risk to your baby, and it will require immediate attention.

HOW TO READ A
NUTRITION LABEL

You've seen nutrition labels countless times on packaged food products, but do you know what to look for or how to make sense of a nutrition label? Understanding how to decode a nutrition label will help you make better food decisions that improve your diabetes management. With so many food options at the supermarket, it can quickly get confusing to know what to choose. In 2016, the FDA announced a new Nutrition Facts label for packaged foods that would make it easier for consumers to make informed choices. They updated the label to reflect new scientific information. Other changes in the label include: added sugars, larger size of the calories label, and simplifying how portion sizes are determined.

Decoding a Nutrition Label: 11 Key Components

- **Serving size**—The first step in reading a label is noting the serving size. This represents a standard measurement or set amount of food. The nutrition information listed is meant only for that one serving of food. Ideally, the serving size is meant to represent a typical serving of food consumed by most Americans. This is a new update from previous labels. The font size of the serving is also larger and easier to read. Keep in mind, not all packages are the same, so the serving size might be different than the amount you are accustomed to eating or different than what your healthcare team recommends.

- **Servings per container**—This is how many servings are included in the entire food package or container. Take, for example, a gallon of milk. The serving size is usually 8 oz. So, the servings per container are 16.

- **Calories**—Calories provide us with energy or fuel for our bodies. During pregnancy, you will need about 300 extra calories in the second and third trimesters. But we want to be mindful of consuming the appropriate number of calories our bodies need. We know that consuming too many calories is linked to

Nutrition Facts

4 servings per container
Serving size 1 1/2 cup (208g)

Amount per serving
Calories 240

	% Daily Value*
Total Fat 4g	**5%**
Saturated Fat 1.5g	**8%**
Trans Fat 0g	
Cholesterol 5mg	**2%**
Sodium 430mg	**19%**
Total Carbohydrate 46g	**17%**
Dietary Fiber 7g	**25%**
Total Sugars 4g	
Includes 2g Added Sugars	**4%**
Protein 11g	
Vitamin D 2mcg	10%
Calcium 260mg	20%
Iron 6mg	35%
Potassium 240mg	6%

* The % Daily Value (DV) tells you how much a nutrient in a serving of food contributes to a daily diet. 2,000 calories a day is used for general nutrition advice.

FDA website

obesity and being overweight. It's not expected for you to count calories, nor should you be afraid of calories. Just be mindful. You may want to avoid very high-calorie foods with minimal nutrition. Instead, choose nutrient-dense foods like fresh vegetables and fruits, whole grains, and lean meats.

- **Total Carbohydrate—** An important component not to be overlooked by people with diabetes. Total carbohydrate includes sugar, fiber, and other starches. It's essential you use the total carbohydrate measurement when counting carbohydrates, and not the count specifically for sugars as this is already calculated in total carbohydrate.

- **Added Sugars—** Added sugars include things like table sugar, honey, syrup, or other forms of sugar from concentrated fruit or vegetable juices. The recommendation is to limit added sugars to no more than 10% of our total calorie intake. The new FDA label requires that added sugars be included in all labels and that it is included in the total carbohydrate amount. Added sugars are not meant to be confused with natural sources of sugar like fruits (fructose) or milk (lactose). In the case of diabetes, it is accounted for in total carbohydrates. Essentially, the less added sugar, the better.

- **Dietary Fiber—** The more fiber, the better. Fiber will help digestion and delay spikes in blood glucose. Look for foods with 3 g fiber or more. Pregnant women need 28 g of fiber a day.

- **Sugar Alcohols—** A type of carbohydrate that is usually added as a sweetener to lower-sugar products as it has about half the calories of regular sugar. This is not to be confused with a non-nutritive sweetener like aspartame, sucralose, or others as these have no carbs or sugar. Commonly used sugar alcohols include maltitol and sorbitol. Side effects of sugar alcohols include diarrhea, cramps, and gastrointestinal discomfort.

- **Total Fat/Saturated Fat/Trans Fat—** Health experts recommend limiting saturated fat, trans fat, and cholesterol as much as possible. Keep in mind that total fat will include all types of fat, including healthy monounsaturated and polyunsaturated fats (like those found in avocados, nuts, and seeds). Look for mono and poly fats instead of saturated and trans.

- **Sodium**—We know excess sodium intake is linked with high blood pressure. Being overweight and having diabetes in pregnancy increase your risk of developing preeclampsia, so it will be important to keep track of your sodium consumption to help manage your blood pressure. Choose foods that are lower in sodium. Watch out for things like sauces, frozen foods, and highly processed foods. One teaspoon of salt = 2,300 mg sodium.
- **Ingredients**—The ingredients are listed in descending order by weight, starting with the primary or heaviest ingredients first. You want to look for whole, nutritious ingredients such as whole grains, healthy fats, and real fruits and vegetables.
- **%DV**—Daily values (DV) show the percentage of each nutrient based on a 2,000-calorie diet. They can be a good reference point to compare one food to the other when serving sizes are similar. You want to aim for high %DV of calcium, fiber, and vitamins A, D, and C; look for a low %DV for sodium, cholesterol, saturated fat, and added sugars.

BEST SNACKS FOR PREGNANCY

W ho doesn't love a good snack? There is no question that we are a snack-loving nation, and the $27 billion spent a year on snacks in the U.S. proves it. But snacks do have a purpose in our lives. Nutritionally speaking, snacks will help you maintain stable blood glucose, meet important nutrient requirements, keep hunger at bay, and provide extra nutrition for your growing baby. When you have diabetes, the type of snack as well as the timing will be very important to track.

Reasons to Snack
- Help you keep full longer
- Meet nutritional needs
- Complement nutrition obtained from regular meals

- Help stabilize blood glucose
- Avoid low blood glucose while keeping you from getting too hungry.

Depending on your needs and blood glucose control, you might require 1–3 snacks a day. These snacks can range from 5–25 g carbohydrate. It will depend on your blood glucose level, individualized meal plan, and carbohydrate goals. When choosing a snack, I recommend following the "FFP" rule: fat, fiber, and protein. Including snacks that have one of these three things will help you keep stable blood glucose and help satisfy your hunger by making you feel full longer.

On the next page are nutritious and hearty snacks that will keep you feeling satisfied and happy until the next meal (Table 27.1). If you are on insulin or find that your blood glucose is higher after meals, and it's harder to consume snacks with 15–25 g of carbohydrates, there is a selection of lower-carbs snacks with 5–10 g carbohydrate, which will prevent spikes in blood glucose.

Mix and match items in Table 27.1, making sure you choose your favorite combination that includes FFP.

TABLE 27.1 Mix-and-Match Snacks to Meet FFP Rule

		Calories	Carbs
Fiber	1 cup air-popped popcorn	30	6
	4 Triscuits	80	13
	1/2 cup fresh raspberries	32	7
	1/2 cup fresh blueberries	42	11
	1/2 medium apple	47	12
	1/2 red bell pepper	18	4
	1 cup sliced cucumber (10–15 slices)	14	2.5
	1 stalk celery	6	1
	8 baby carrots	32	8
	1/4 cup pomegranate arils	36	8
	1/2 English muffin	65	13
	1 graham cracker (large rectangle/2 squares)	60	10
	1 cup steamed edamame (in pods)	113	8
Fat	1/2 oz almonds (about 10 almonds)	84	2
	1/4 avocado	55	3
	2 Tbsp light cream cheese	60	2
	1 Tbsp peanut butter	95	3.5
	2 Tbsp hummus	52	6
	2 Tbsp ranch dressing	130	2
Protein	1 oz pistachios, in shell	85	4
	1 low-fat string cheese	80	1
	1 hard-boiled egg	78	0
	1/4 cup tuna salad	115	2
	1 oz reduced-fat cheese	50	0.5
	1/2 cup low-fat cottage cheese	81	3
	1/2 cup nonfat plain Greek yogurt	72	4.5
	2 oz smoked salmon	100	1

Hearty Snacks

Quick-and-easy ideas for larger snacks or smaller meals.

Snack #1
(180 calories, 25 g carbohydrate)
- 1 (6-inch) whole-wheat tortilla
- 2 Tbsp hummus
- 1/2 cup bell pepper strips
- 1 cup baby spinach

Snack #2
(210 calories, 20 g carbohydrate)
- 1 slice whole-wheat toast
- 1 large slice tomato
- 1/4 avocado, sliced
- 1 tsp olive oil
- 1/4 cup sliced cucumber
- Salt and pepper

Snack #3
(210 calories, 17 g carbohydrate)
- 1 small, whole-wheat dinner roll
- 1/2 oz cheddar cheese
- 2 pieces leaf lettuce
- 1 tsp Dijon or other mustard
- 2 oz sliced turkey

Snack #4
(130 calories, 20 g carbohydrate)
- 1 small, whole-wheat dinner roll
- 1 Tbsp herb cream cheese
- 1/2 cup baby spinach

- 1/4 cup sliced cucumber
- 1/4 avocado, sliced

Snack #5
(220 calories, 23 g carbohydrate)
- 1/2 whole-grain pita
- 1/2 cup arugula or spinach
- 1 Tbsp crumbled feta cheese
- 1 jarred roasted red pepper, sliced
- 3 Kalamata olives, chopped
- 1 tsp olive oil

Snack #6
(180 calories, 19 g carbohydrate)
- 1 (6-inch) whole-wheat tortilla
- 1/4 cup reduced-fat shredded cheddar cheese
- 2 Tbsp salsa
- 1/4 cup Plain Greek yogurt

Snack #7
(160 calories, 22 g carbohydrate)
  Berry smoothie made with:
- 1/2 cup frozen mixed berries
- 1/4 small banana
- 1/4 cup plain Greek yogurt
- 2 Tbsp ground flaxseed

Snack #8
(200 calories, 24 g carbohydrate)
- 1 corn tostada
- 1/4 avocado, diced
- 2 Tbsp salsa
- 1/4 cup black beans

Snack #9
(180 calories, 17 g carbohydrate)
Yogurt parfait made with:
- 1/2 cup frozen mixed berries
- 1/2 cup plain Greek yogurt
- 2 Tbsp slivered almonds

Snack #10
(220 calories, 20 g carbohydrate)
- 1 slice whole-wheat bread
- 2 Tbsp light cream cheese
- 1/2 tsp agave nectar
- 5 walnut halves

Snack #11
(150 calories, 18 g carbohydrate)
- 1 slice rye bread
- 2 Tbsp light cream cheese
- 1/4 cup sliced cucumbers
- 2 tsp fresh dill (or 1/2 tsp dried dill)

Low-Carb Snacks

(Less than 5 g carbohydrate)
- 1 oz nuts (about 1 handful)
- 2 Tbsp regular peanut/almond butter with 1/2 cup celery
- 1 cup popcorn
- Tomato and mozzarella skewers
- Sugar-free gelatin dessert
- Cheese and ham rolls
- 1 cup broccoli with low-fat ranch dressing
- 1/2 cup cottage cheese
- Mini egg frittatas
- Cucumber/tomato salad with lemon, olive oil, and feta

chapter 28

MEAL PLANS AND
TASTY RECIPES

Visit goodlifediabetes.com/recipes
or diabetesfoodhub.org

Meal Plans

DAY 1 1,800-Calorie Meal Plan (Recipes in bold can be found on pages 292–318)

Meal	Food & Portion Size	Calories	CHO (g)	Total Cals	Total CHO (g)	Carb Choices
BREAKFAST	1 slice whole-grain toast	82	14			
	2 eggs, scrambled	180	1	297	17	1
	2 Tbsp salsa	10	2			
	2 Tbsp reduced-fat shredded cheese	25	0			
SNACK	15 grapes	52	13	94	15	1
	1/2 oz pistachios (in shell)	42	2			
LUNCH	1 6-inch whole-wheat tortilla	100	15			
Hummus Wrap	2 Tbsp hummus	53	6			
	1/4 avocado, sliced	55	3			
	1 cup mixed lettuce	6	1			
	1/4 cup garbanzo beans	67	11	450	45	3
	1 Tbsp pepitas (shelled pumpkin seeds)	42	1			
	1 tsp olive oil	39	0			
	1/2 cup plain nonfat Greek yogurt	72	5			
	1/4 cup raspberries	16	4			

SNACK	3 cups air-popped popcorn	90	18	172	20	1.5
	1/2 cup cucumber slices	7	1			
	1 Tbsp ranch dressing	75	1			
DINNER	**Grilled Salmon with Mango and Tomato Salad**	220	10			
	Cilantro Lime Quinoa	145	22	575	40	3
	2 cups mixed lettuce	12	2			
	1/2 cup cherry tomatoes	13	3			
	2 Tbsp reduced fat shredded cheese	25	0			
	1 Tbsp balsamic vinaigrette	80	1			
	1/2-oz square dark chocolate	80	2			
PM SNACK	**1/3 cup Chunky Pistachio Granola**	120	13	192	18	1
	1/2 cup nonfat plain greek yogurt	72	5			
	DAILY TOTALS			1780	155	

257

DAY 1 2,000-Calorie Meal Plan

Meal	Food & Portion Size	Calories	CHO (g)	Total Cals	Total CHO (g)	Carb Choices
BREAKFAST	1 slice whole-grain toast	82	14			
	2 eggs, scrambled	180	1			
	2 Tbsp salsa	10	2	437	31	2
	2 Tbsp reduced-fat shredded cheese	25	0			
	2 slices turkey bacon	80	0			
	1 cup diced peaches (or 1 peach)	60	14			
SNACK	15 grapes	52	13	94	15	1
	1/2 oz pistachios (in shell)	42	2			
LUNCH	1 6-inch whole-wheat tortilla	100	15			
Hummus Wrap	2 Tbsp hummus	53	6			
	1/4 avocado, sliced	55	3			
	1 cup mixed lettuce	6	1			
	1/4 cup garbanzo beans	67	11	525	54	3.5
	1 Tbsp pepitas (shelled pumpkin seeds)	42	1			
	1 tsp olive oil	39	0			
	1/2 cup plain nonfat Greek yogurt	72	5			
	1/4 cup raspberries	16	4			
	2 No-Bake Peanut Butter and Chocolate Bites	75	9			

SNACK	3 cups air-popped popcorn	90	18		
	1/2 cup cucumber slices	7	1	172	20	1.5
	1 Tbsp ranch dressing	75	1		
DINNER	**Grilled Salmon with Mango and Tomato Salad**	220	10		
	Cilantro Lime Quinoa	145	22		
	2 cups mixed lettuce	12	2		
	1/2 cup cherry tomatoes	13	3	575	40	3
	2 Tbsp reduced-fat shredded cheese	25	0		
	1 Tbsp balsamic vinaigrette	80	1		
	1/2-oz square dark chocolate	80	2		
PM SNACK	**1/3 cup Chunky Pistachio Granola**	120	13	192	18	1
	1/2 cup plain nonfat Greek yogurt	72	5		
	DAILY TOTALS			1995	178	

259

DAY 1 2,200-Calorie Meal Plan

Meal	Food & Portion Size	Calories	CHO (g)	Total Cals	Total CHO (g)	Carb Choices
BREAKFAST	1 slice whole-grain toast	82	14	552	31	3
	3 eggs, scrambled	270	1			
	2 Tbsp salsa	10	2			
	1/4 cup reduced-fat shredded cheese	50	0			
	2 slices turkey bacon	80	0			
	1 cup diced peaches (or 1 peach)	60	14			
SNACK	15 grapes	52	13	136	17	1
	1 oz pistachios (in shell)	84	4			
LUNCH	1 6-inch whole-wheat tortilla	100	15	525	54	3.5
Hummus Wrap	2 Tbsp hummus	53	6			
	1/4 avocado, sliced	55	3			
	1 cup mixed lettuce	6	1			
	1/4 cup garbanzo beans	67	11			
	1 Tbsp pepitas (shelled pumpkin seeds)	42	1			
	1 tsp olive oil	39	0			
	1/2 cup plain nonfat Greek yogurt	72	5			
	1/4 cup raspberries	16	4			
	2 No-Bake Peanut Butter and Chocolate Bites	75	9			

SNACK	3 cups air-popped popcorn	90	18	172	20	1.5
	1/2 cup cucumber slices	7	1			
	1 Tbsp ranch dressing	75	1			
DINNER	**Grilled Salmon with Mango and tomato salad**	220	10	575	40	3
	Cilantro Lime Quinoa	145	22			
	2 cups mixed lettuce	12	2			
	1/2 cup cherry tomatoes	13	3			
	2 Tbsp reduced fat shredded cheese	25	0			
	1 Tbsp balsamic vinaigrette	80	1			
	1/2-oz square dark chocolate	80	2			
PM SNACK	**1/3 cup Chunky Pistachio Granola**	120	13	264	22	1.5
	1 cup plain nonfat Greek Yogurt	144	9			
	DAILY TOTALS			2224	184	

261

DAY 2 1,800-Calorie Meal Plan

Meal	Food & Portion Size	Calories	CHO (g)	Total Cals	Total CHO (g)	Carb Choices
BREAKFAST	Overnight Quinoa	360	32	360	32	2
SNACK	3/4 cup tomato soup	78	12	138	22	1.5
	1/2 oz whole-grain crackers	60	10			
LUNCH	Bento Box	480	55	480	55	3.5
SNACK	Cucumber Gucamole	45	4	115	14	1
	1/2 oz corn tortilla chips	70	10			
DINNER	Open-Face Turkey Burger	320	18	532	44	3
	Sweet Potato Fries	130	24			
	1/2 cup sliced cucumber	7	1			
	1 Tbsp ranch dressing	75	1			
PM SNACK	Greek Yogurt Chocolate Mousse	130	17	130	17	1
	DAILY TOTALS			1755	184	

DAY 2 2,000-Calorie Meal Plan

Meal	Food & Portion Size	Calories	CHO (g)	Total Cals	Total CHO (g)	Carb Choices
BREAKFAST	Overnight Quinoa	360	32	360	32	2
SNACK	3/4 cup tomato soup	78	12			
	1/2 oz whole grain crackers	60	10	188	22	1.5
	1 oz reduced-fat cheese	50	0			
LUNCH	Bento Box	480	55	512	62	4
	1/2 cup raspberries	32	7			
SNACK	Cucumber Gucamole	45	4	185	23	1.5
	1 oz corn tortilla chips	140	19			
DINNER	Open-Face Turkey Burger	320	18			
	Sweet Potato Fries	130	24	532	44	3
	1/2 cup sliced cucumber	7	1			
	1 Tbsp ranch dressing	75	1			
PM SNACK	Greek Yogurt Chocolate Mousse	130	17	163	18	1
	1 Tbsp sliced almonds	33	1			
	DAILY TOTALS			1940	201	

263

DAY 2 2,200-Calorie Meal Plan

Meal	Food & Portion Size	Calories	CHO (g)	Total Cals	Total CHO (g)	Carb Choices
BREAKFAST	**Overnight Quinoa**	360	32	360	32	2
SNACK	3/4 cup tomato soup	78	12	188	22	1.5
	1/2 ounce whole grain crackers	60	10			
	1 oz reduced-fat cheese	50	0			
LUNCH	**Bento Box**	480	55	593	65	4
	1/2 cup raspberries	32	7			
	1/2 cup low-fat cottage cheese	81	3			
SNACK	**Cucumber Gucamole**	45	4	185	23	1.5
	1 oz corn tortilla chips	140	19			
DINNER	**Open-Face Turkey Burger**	320	18	532	44	3
	Sweet Potato Fries	130	24			
	1/2 cup sliced cucumber	7	1			
	1 Tbsp ranch dressing	75	1			
PM SNACK	**Greek Yogurt Chocolate Mousse**	130	17	196	18	1
	2 Tbsp sliced almonds	66	1			
	DAILY TOTALS			2054	204	

DAY 3 1,800-Calorie Meal Plan

Meal	Food & Portion Size	Calories	CHO (g)	Total Cals	Total CHO (g)	Carb Choices
BREAKFAST	**Herbed Soft Scrambled–Eggs on Toast**	170	16	285	33	2
	1/4 avocado	55	3			
	1 cup diced peaches (or 1 peach)	60	14			
SNACK	1/2 cup sliced cucumber	7	1	164	24	1.5
	1/2 cup plain nonfat Greek yogurt	72	5			
	1/2 whole-grain pita	85	18			
LUNCH	**Mason Jar Salad**	460	38	535	47	3
	2 No-Bake Peanut Butter and Chocolate Bites	75	9			
SNACK	**Zucchini and Date Muffin**	145	21	225	22	1.5
	1 low-fat string cheese	80	1			
DINNER	**2 Pork Tacos**	260	26	448	48	3
	1/2 cup black beans	110	19			
	2 Tbsp salsa	10	2			
	1/4 cup reduced-fat shredded cheese	50	0			
	2 Tbsp plain nonfat Greek yogurt	18	1			
PM SNACK	1 Tbsp peanut butter	95	4	160	17	1
	1/2 English muffin	65	13			
	DAILY TOTALS			1817	191	

DAY 3 2,000-Calorie Meal Plan

Meal	Food & Portion Size	Calories	CHO (g)	Total Cals	Total CHO (g)	Carb Choices
BREAKFAST	**Herbed Soft Scrambled–Eggs on Toast**	170	16	285	33	2
	1/4 avocado	55	3			
	1 cup diced peaches (or 1 peach)	60	14			
SNACK	1/2 cup sliced cucumber	7	1	164	24	1.5
	1/2 cup plain nonfat Greek yogurt	72	5			
	1/2 whole-grain pita	85	18			
LUNCH	**Mason Jar Salad**	460	38	535	47	3
	2 No-Bake Peanut Butter and Chocolate Bites	75	9			
SNACK	**Zucchini and Date Muffin**	145	21	257	28	2
	1 low-fat string cheese	80	1			
	1/2 cup sliced strawberries	27	6			

DINNER						
2 Pork Tacos	260	26	558	54	3.5
1/2 cup black beans	110	19			
2 Tbsp salsa	10	2			
1/4 cup reduced-fat shredded cheese	50	0			
2 Tbsp plain nonfat Greek yogurt	18	1			
1/2 avocado	110	6			
PM SNACK					
1 Tbsp peanut butter	95	4	187	23	1.5
1/2 English muffin	65	13			
1/2 cup sliced strawberries	27	6			
DAILY TOTALS			1986	210	

DAY 3 2,200-Calorie Meal Plan

Meal	Food & Portion Size	Calories	CHO (g)	Total Cals	Total CHO (g)	Carb Choices
BREAKFAST	**Herbed Soft Scrambled–Eggs on Toast**	170	16	453	37	2.5
	1/4 avocado	55	3			
	1 cup diced peaches (or 1 peach)	60	14			
	1 oz almonds (about 20 almonds)	168	4			
SNACK	1/2 cup sliced cucumber	7	1	164	24	1.5
	1/2 cup plain nonfat Greek yogurt	72	5			
	1/2 whole-grain pita	85	18			
LUNCH	**Mason Jar Salad**	460	38	535	47	3
	2 No-Bake Peanut Butter and Chocolate Bites	75	9			
SNACK	**Zucchini and Date Muffin**	145	21	257	28	2
	1 low-fat string cheese	80	1			
	1/2 cup sliced strawberries	27	6			

DINNER					
2 Pork Tacos	260	26	558	54	3.5
1/2 cup black beans	110	19			
2 Tbsp salsa	10	2			
1/4 cup reduced-fat shredded cheese	50	0			
2 Tbsp plain nonfat Greek yogurt	18	1			
1/2 avocado	110	6			
PM SNACK					
1 Tbsp peanut butter	95	4	214	29	2
1/2 English muffin	65	13			
1 cup sliced strawberries	54	12			
DAILY TOTALS			**2181**	**219**	

DAY 4 1,800-Calorie Meal Plan

Meal	Food & Portion Size	Calories	CHO (g)	Total Cals	Total CHO (g)	Carb Choices
BREAKFAST	Salmon Toast with Greens	310	25	310	25	1.5
SNACK	1 small pear	84	22	126	24	1.5
	1/2 oz pistachios	42	2			
LUNCH	2 Pork Tacos	260	26	448	48	3
	1/2 cup black beans	110	19			
	2 Tbsp salsa	10	2			
	1/4 cup reduced fat shredded cheese	50	0			
	2 Tbsp plain nonfat Greek yogurt	18	1			
SNACK	Cucumber Guacamole	45	4	115	14	1
	1/2 ounce corn tortilla chips	70	10			
DINNER	Open-Face Turkey Burger	320	18	605	49	3
	Sweet Potato Fries	130	24			
	2 cups mixed lettuce	12	2			
	1/2 cup cherry tomatoes	13	3			
	2 Tbsp ranch dressing	130	2			
PM SNACK	1 apple	90	20	186	24	1.5
	1 Tbsp nut butter	96	4			
	DAILY TOTALS			1790	184	

DAY 4 2,000-Calorie Meal Plan

Meal	Food & Portion Size	Calories	CHO (g)	Total Cals	Total CHO (g)	Carb Choices
BREAKFAST	**Salmon Toast with Greens**	310	25	342	32	2
	1/2 cup raspberries	32	7			
SNACK	1 small pear	84	22	126	24	1.5
	1/2 oz pistachios	42	2			
LUNCH	**2 Pork Tacos**	260	26	558	54	3.5
	1/2 cup black beans	110	19			
	2 Tbsp salsa	10	2			
	1/4 cup reduced-fat shredded cheese	50	0			
	2 Tbsp plain nonfat Greek yogurt	18	1			
	1/2 avocado	110	6			
SNACK	**Cucumber Guacamole**	45	4	185	23	1.5
	1 oz corn tortilla chips	140	19			
DINNER	**Open-Face Turkey Burger**	320	18	605	49	3
	Sweet Potato Fries	130	24			
	2 cups mixed lettuce	12	2			
	1/2 cup cherry tomatoes	13	3			
	2 Tbsp ranch dressing	130	2			
PM SNACK	1 apple	90	20	186	24	1.5
	1 Tbsp nut butter	96	4			
	DAILY TOTALS			2002	206	

271

DAY 4 2,200-Calorie Meal Plan

Meal	Food & Portion Size	Calories	CHO (g)	Total Cals	Total CHO (g)	Carb Choices
BREAKFAST	**Salmon Toast with Greens**	310	25			
	1/2 cup raspberries	32	7	480	39	2.5
	2 Tbsp sliced almonds	66	2			
	1/2 cup plain nonfat Greek yogurt	72	5			
SNACK	1 small pear	84	22	168	24	1.5
	1 oz pistachios	84	2			
LUNCH	**2 Pork Tacos**	260	26			
	1/2 cup black beans	110	19			
	2 Tbsp salsa	10	2	558	54	3.5
	1/4 cup reduced-fat shredded cheese	50	0			
	2 Tbsp plain nonfat Greek yogurt	18	1			
	1/2 avocado	110	6			

SNACK	**Cucumber Guacamole**	45	4	185	23	1.5
	1 oz corn tortilla chips	140	19			
DINNER	**Open-Face Turkey Burger**	320	18			
	Sweet Potato Fries	130	24			
	2 cups mixed lettuce	12	2	605	49	3
	1/2 cup cherry tomatoes	13	3			
	2 Tbsp ranch dressing	130	2			
PM SNACK	1 apple	90	20	186	24	1.5
	1 Tbsp nut butter	96	4			
	DAILY TOTALS			2182	213	

273

DAY 5 1,800-Calorie Meal Plan

Meal	Food & Portion Size	Calories	CHO (g)	Total Cals	Total CHO (g)	Carb Choices
BREAKFAST	**Breakfast Taco**	370	30	450	32	2
	2 slices turkey bacon	80	2			
SNACK	1/2 cup low-fat cottage cheese	81	3	135	15	1
	1 cup sliced strawberries	54	12			
LUNCH	**Mason Jar Salad**	460	38	592	53	3.5
	1 low-fat string cheese	80	1			
	1/2 cup seedless grapes	52	14			
SNACK	1 cup carrots	50	12	103	18	1
	2 Tbsp hummus	53	6			
DINNER	**Chicken Chili**	290	23	358	24	1.5
	2 Tbsp plain nonfat Greek yogurt	18	1			
	1/4 cup reduced-fat shredded cheese	50	0			
PM SNACK	**Dark Chocolate–Covered Strawberries**	140	14	140	14	1
	DAILY TOTALS			1778	156	

DAY 5 2,000-Calorie Meal Plan

Meal	Food & Portion Size	Calories	CHO (g)	Total Cals	Total CHO (g)	Carb Choices
BREAKFAST	**Breakfast Taco**	370	30	**450**	**32**	2
	2 slices turkey bacon	80	2			
SNACK	1/2 cup low-fat cottage cheese	81	3	**235**	**17**	1
	1 cup sliced strawberries	54	12			
	1/2 oz walnuts (about 6-7 halves)	100	2			
LUNCH	**Mason Jar Salad**	460	38	**592**	**53**	3.5
	1 low-fat string cheese	80	1			
	1/2 cup seedless grapes	52	14			
SNACK	1 cup carrots	50	12	**103**	**18**	1
	2 Tbsp hummus	53	6			
DINNER	**Chicken Chili**	290	23	**358**	**24**	1.5
	2 Tbsp plain nonfat Greek yogurt	18	1			
	1/4 cup reduced-fat shredded cheese	50	0			
PM SNACK	**Dark Chocolate-Covered Strawberries**	140	14	**221**	**17**	1.5
	1/2 cup low-fat cottage cheese	81	3			
	DAILY TOTALS			1959	161	

DAY 5 2,200-Calorie Meal Plan

Meal	Food & Portion Size	Calories	CHO (g)	Total Cals	Total CHO (g)	Carb Choices
BREAKFAST	**Breakfast Taco**	370	30	540	52	3.5
	2 slices turkey bacon	80	2			
	1 small apple	90	20			
SNACK	1/2 cup low-fat cottage cheese	81	3	235	17	1
	1 cup sliced strawberries	54	12			
	1/2 oz walnuts (about 6-7 halves)	100	2			
LUNCH	**Mason Jar Salad**	460	38	644	67	3.5
	1 low-fat string cheese	80	1			
	1 cup seedless grapes	104	28			
SNACK	1 cup carrots	50	12	103	18	1
	2 Tbsp hummus	53	6			
DINNER	**Chicken Chili**	290	23	428	34	2
	2 Tbsp plain nonfat Greek yogurt	18	1			
	1/4 cup reduced-fat shredded cheese	50	0			
	1/2 oz corn tortilla chips	70	10			
PM SNACK	**Dark Chocolate–Covered Strawberries**	140	14	221	17	1.5
	1/2 cup low-fat cottage cheese	81	3			
	DAILY TOTALS			2171	205	

DAY 6 1,800-Calorie Meal Plan

Meal	Food & Portion Size	Calories	CHO (g)	Total Cals	Total CHO (g)	Carb Choices
BREAKFAST	1 cup nonfat plain Greek yogurt	144	9	446	42	2.5
	1/2 cup Chunky Pistachio Granola	185	22			
	1/2 cup raspberries	32	7			
	1 oz pistachios (in shell)	85	4			
SNACK	15 grapes	52	14	132	15	1
	1 low-fat string cheese	80	1			
LUNCH	**Chicken Chili**	290	23	328	28	2
	1/4 cup salsa	20	4			
	2 Tbsp plain nonfat Greek yogurt	18	1			
	1/4 cup reduced-fat shredded cheese	50	0			
SNACK	2 Tbsp hummus	53	6	142	25	1.5
	1/2 whole-grain pita	85	18			
	1/4 cup sliced cucumber	4	1			
DINNER	**Baked Lemon-Mustard Sheet Pan Salmon**	370	28	515	46	3
	Easy Caprese Salad	70	4			
	1 small whole-wheat dinner roll	75	14			
PM SNACK	**Cucumber Guacamole**	45	4	115	14	1
	1/2 oz corn tortilla chips	70	10			
	DAILY TOTALS			1728	170	

DAY 6 2,000-Calorie Meal Plan

Meal	Food & Portion Size	Calories	CHO (g)	Total Cals	Total CHO (g)	Carb Choices
BREAKFAST	1 cup nonfat plain Greek yogurt	144	9			
	1/2 cup Chunky Pistachio Granola	185	22	**446**	**42**	**2.5**
	1/2 cup raspberries	32	7			
	1 oz pistachios (in shell)	85	4			
SNACK	15 grapes	52	14	**132**	**15**	**1**
	1 low-fat string cheese	80	1			
LUNCH	**Chicken Chili**	290	23			
	1/4 cup salsa	20	4			
	2 Tbsp plain nonfat Greek yogurt	18	1			
	1/4 cup reduced-fat shredded cheese	50	0	**533**	**35**	**2.6**
	2 cups mixed lettuce	12	2			
	1/2 cup cherry tomatoes	13	3			
	2 Tbsp ranch dressing	130	2			

SNACK	2 Tbsp hummus	53	6			
	1/2 whole-grain pita	85	18	142	25	1.5
	1/4 cup sliced cucumber	4	1			
DINNER	Baked Lemon-Mustard Sheet Pan Salmon	370	28			
	Easy Caprese Salad	70	4	515	46	3
	1 small whole-wheat dinner roll	75	14			
PM SNACK	Cucumber Guacamole	45	4	185	23	1.5
	1 oz corn tortilla chips	140	19			
	DAILY TOTALS			1953	186	

279

DAY 6 2,200-Calorie Meal Plan

Meal	Food & Portion Size	Calories	CHO (g)	Total Cals	Total CHO (g)	Carb Choices
BREAKFAST	1 cup plain nonfat greek yogurt	144	9			
	1/2 cup Chunky Pistachio Granola	185	22	478	49	3
	1 cup raspberries	64	14			
	1 oz pistachios (in shell)	85	4			
SNACK	15 grapes	52	14			
	1 low-fat string cheese	80	1	232	17	1
	1/2 oz walnuts (about 6-7 halves)	100	2			
LUNCH	**Chicken Chili**	290	23			
	1/4 cup salsa	20	4			
	2 Tbsp plain nonfat Greek yogurt	18	1			
	1/4 cup reduced-fat shredded cheese	50	0	533	35	2
	2 cups mixed lettuce	12	2			
	1/2 cup cherry tomatoes	13	3			
	2 Tbsp ranch dressing	130	2			

SNACK	1/4 cup hummus	106	12		
	1/2 whole-grain pita	85	18	195	31	2
	1/4 cup sliced cucumber	4	1		
DINNER	**Baked Lemon-Mustard Sheet Pan Salmon**	370	28		
	Easy Caprese Salad	70	4	515	46	3
	1 small whole-wheat dinner roll	75	14		
PM SNACK	**Cucumber Guacamole**	45	4	185	23	1.5
	1 oz corn tortilla chips	140	19		
	DAILY TOTALS		2138		201

281

DAY 7 1,800-Calorie Meal Plan

Meal	Food & Portion Size	Calories	CHO (g)	Total Cals	Total CHO (g)	Carb Choices
BREAKFAST	**Simple Sweet Potato Pancakes**	200	28	494	47	3
	2 Tbsp peanut butter	190	7			
	1/2 cup fresh raspberries	32	7			
	1/2 cup plain nonfat Greek yogurt	72	5			
SNACK	8 baby carrots	32	8	85	14	1
	2 Tbsp hummus	53	6			
LUNCH	**Avocado Egg Toast**	240	16	400	40	1.5
	Easy Caprese Salad	70	4			
	1 small apple	90	20			
SNACK	2 cups air-popped popcorn	60	12	144	14	1
	1/2 oz almonds (about 10 almonds)	84	2			

DINNER	**Crock Pot Chicken Cacciatore**	170	18			
	1/2 cup cooked whole-wheat pasta	119	24			
	2 cups mixed lettuce	16	3	528	50	3.5
	1/2 cup cherry tomatoes	13	3			
	1/4 cup reduced-fat shredded cheese	50	0			
	2 Tbsp balsamic vinaigrette	160	2			
PM SNACK	**2 No-Bake Peanut Butter and Chocolate Bites**	75	9	155	10	1
	1 low-fat string cheese	80	1			
	DAILY TOTALS			1806	175	

283

DAY 7 2,000-Calorie Meal Plan

Meal	Food & Portion Size	Calories	CHO (g)	Total Cals	Total CHO (g)	Carb Choices
BREAKFAST	**Simple Sweet Potato Pancakes**	200	28	494	47	3
	2 Tbsp peanut butter	190	7			
	1/2 cup fresh raspberries	32	7			
	1/2 cup plain nonfat Greek yogurt	72	5			
SNACK	8 baby carrots	32	8	145	24	1.5
	2 Tbsp hummus	53	6			
	1/2 oz whole-grain crackers	60	10			
LUNCH	**Avocado Egg Toast**	240	16	400	40	1.5
	Easy Caprese Salad	70	4			
	1 small apple	90	20			
SNACK	2 cups air-popped popcorn	60	12	144	14	1
	1/2 oz almonds (about 10 almonds)	84	2			

DINNER	**Crock Pot Chicken Cacciatore**	170	18			
	1/2 cup cooked whole-wheat pasta	119	24			
	2 cups mixed lettuce	16	3			
	1/2 cup cherry tomatoes	13	3	583	53	3.5
	1/4 cup reduced-fat shredded cheese	50	0			
	2 Tbsp balsamic vinaigrette	160	2			
	1/4 avocado	55	3			
PM SNACK	**3 No-Bake Peanut Butter and Chocolate Bites**	110	13	190	14	1.5
	1 low-fat string cheese	80	1			
	DAILY TOTALS			1956	192	

DAY 7 2,200-Calorie Meal Plan

Meal	Food & Portion Size	Calories	CHO (G)	Total Cals	Total CHO (G)	Carb Choices
BREAKFAST	**Simple Sweet Potato Pancakes**	200	28	560	49	3
	2 Tbsp peanut butter	190	7			
	1/2 cup fresh raspberries	32	7			
	1/2 cup plain nonfat Greek yogurt	72	5			
	2 Tbsp sliced almonds	66	2			
SNACK	8 baby carrots	32	8	198	30	2
	1/4 cup hummus	106	12			
	1/2 oz whole-grain crackers	60	10			
LUNCH	**Avocado Egg Toast**	240	16	400	40	1.5
	Easy Caprese Salad	70	4			
	1 small apple	90	20			
SNACK	3 cups air-popped popcorn	90	18	258	22	1.5
	1 oz almonds (about 20 almonds)	168	4			

DINNER	Crock Pot Chicken Cacciatore	170	18			
	1/2 cup cooked whole-wheat pasta	119	24			
	2 cups mixed lettuce	16	3			
	1/2 cup cherry tomatoes	13	3	583	53	3.5
	1/4 cup reduced-fat shredded cheese	50	0			
	2 Tbsp balsamic vinaigrette	160	2			
	1/4 avocado	55	3			
PM SNACK	3 No-Bake Peanut Butter and Chocolate Bites	110	13	190	14	1.5
	1 low-fat string cheese	80	1			
	DAILY TOTALS			2189	208	

287

Hearty Snacks
Quick-and-Easy Ideas for Larger Snacks or Small Meals

Food & Portion Size	Calories	Carbs (g)	Total Calories	Total Carbs (g)
1 (6-inch) whole-wheat tortilla	102	15		
2 Tbsp hummus	53	6		
1/2 cup bell pepper strips	14	3	175	25
1 cup baby spinach	6	1		
1 slice whole-wheat toast	82	14		
1 large slice tomato	5	1		
1/4 avocado, sliced	81	4	212	20
1 tsp olive oil, salt and pepper	40	0		
1/4 cup sliced cucumber	4	1		
1 small whole-wheat dinner roll	75	14		
1/2 oz cheddar cheese	58	1		
2 pieces leaf lettuce	2	0	210	17
1 tsp Dijon or other mustard	5	0		
2 oz sliced turkey	70	2		
1 small whole-wheat dinner roll	75	14		
1 Tbsp herb cream cheese	51	1		
1/2 cup baby spinach	3	1	133	20
1/4 cup sliced cucumber	4	1		
1/4 avocado, sliced	81	4		
1/2 whole-grain pita	85	18		
1/2 cup arugula or spinach	3	0		
1 Tbsp crumbled feta cheese	38	1		
1 jarred roasted red pepper, sliced	10	1	223	23
3 kalamata olives, chopped	47	3		
1 tsp olive oil	40	0		

Food & Portion Size	Calories	Carbs (g)	Total Calories	Total Carbs (g)
1 (6-inch) whole wheat tortilla	102	15		
1/4 cup reduced fat shredded cheddar cheese	50	1	184	19
2 Tbsp salsa	10	2		
plain Greek yogurt	22	1		
Berry Smoothie 1/2 cup frozen mixed berries	50	12		
1/4 small banana	23	6	157	22
1/4 cup plain Greek yogurt	44	2		
2 Tbsp ground flax seed	40	2		
1 corn tostada	58	8		
1/4 avocado, diced	81	4	204	24
2 Tbsp salsa	10	2		
1/4 cup black beans	55	10		
Yogurt Parfait 1/2 cup frozen mixed berries	50	12		
1/2 cup plain Greek yogurt	44	2	180	17
2 Tbsp slivered almonds	86	3		
1 slice whole wheat bread	82	14		
2 Tbsp light cream cheese	60	2	219	20
1/2 tsp agave nectar	11	3		
5 walnut halves	66	1		
1 slice rye bread	83	15		
2 Tbsp light cream cheese	60	2	147	18
sliced cucumber	4	1		
2 tsp fresh or 1/2 tsp dried dill	0	0		

Carb Choice

1 Carb Choice = 15 g of carbohyrate

(Academy of Nutrition and Dietetics; www.eatright.org)

Grains/Breads/Cereals

1 oz bread (for example, 1 slice bread, 1/4 large bagel, or a 6-inch corn tortilla)

1/3 cup cooked rice

1 cup soup

3/4–1 cup cold cereal

1/2 cup cooked cereal

1 small (3-oz) potato

1/2 cup cooked pasta

1/2 English muffin

1 small (6-inch) corn tortilla

1 small (6-inch) flour tortilla or 1/3 of a large 10-inch tortilla

1 small pancake 4 inches long, 1/4-inch thick

Fruits

1 small piece fresh fruit (4 oz)

1/2 cup canned fruit in its own juice (not heavy syrup)

1 cup cantaloupe or honeydew melon

2 Tbsp dried fruit

3 oz grapes (17 small)

1 cup raspberries

3/4 cup blueberries or blackberries

1 1/4 cup strawberries

1/2 grapefruit fresh

1/2 banana or extra small

1/2 small mango or 1/2 cup

1 medium peach

Milk and Yogurt

1 cup low-fat milk

3/4–1 cup plain yogurt or yogurt made with artificial sweetener

1 cup soy milk

Starchy Vegetables

1/2 cup potatoes, green peas, or corn

3 cups raw nonstarchy vegetables

1 1/2 cups cooked nonstarchy vegetables

1/2 cup or (3 1/2 oz) yam/sweet potato

Lentils/Beans

1/2 cup cooked dried beans, lentils, or peas

1/2 cup refried beans canned

1/3 cup baked beans canned

BREAKFAST

Overnight Oats

SERVES: 1
PREP TIME: 5 minutes, plus 6 hours to chil

SERVING SIZE: 1 jar
COOKING TIME: None

INGREDIENTS

1/4 cup rolled oats
1/4 cup skim milk or unsweetened plant-based milk
1 tsp honey
1 tsp chia seeds
1/8 tsp ground cinnamon
PINCH salt (about 1/16 tsp)

Toppings:
1/4 cup blueberries
2 Tbsp chopped walnuts
2 Tbsp low-fat plain Greek yogurt

INSTRUCTIONS

1 Place all ingredients, except toppings, in a mason jar and stir to combine. Cover with lid and refrigerate for at least 6 hours, or overnight.

2 Remove lid, stir again, add toppings, and enjoy.

> NOTE: *Other fruit can be substituted for blueberries, such as pomegranate arils, raspberries, or strawberries. Consider adding 1/8 tsp vanilla extract for even more flavor without additional carbs!*

CHOICES/EXCHANGES: 1 Starch, 1 Carbohydrate, 1 Lean Protein, 2 Fat
BASIC NUTRITIONAL VALUES: **Calories** 280 | Calories from fat 120 | **Total fat** 13.0 g | Saturated fat 1.7 g | Trans fat 0.0 g | **Cholesterol** 15 mg | **Sodium** 180 mg | **Potassium** 330 mg | **Total carbohydrate** 33 g | Dietary fiber 6 g | Sugars 14 g | Added sugars 6 g | **Protein** 11 g | **Phosphorus** 275 mg

Overnight Quinoa

SERVES: 1
PREP TIME: 5 minutes, plus 6 hours to chill

SERVING SIZE: 1 jar
COOKING TIME: None

INGREDIENTS

1/3 cup cooked quinoa

1/4 cup skim milk or unsweetened plant-based milk

2 Tbsp low-fat plain Greek yogurt

1/2 tsp agave nectar

1 tsp chia seeds

1/8 tsp ground cinnamon

PINCH salt (about 1/16 tsp)

Toppings:

1/4 cup blueberries

1 Tbsp peanut butter

2 Tbsp chopped walnuts

INSTRUCTIONS

1 Place all ingredients, except toppings, in a mason jar and stir to combine. Cover with lid and refrigerate for at least 6 hours, or overnight.

2 Remove lid, stir again, add toppings, and enjoy.

NOTE: *Other fruit can be substituted for blueberries, such as pomegranate arils, raspberries, or strawberries. Consider adding 1/8 tsp vanilla extract for even more flavor without additional carbs!*

CHOICES/EXCHANGES: 1 Starch, 1 Carbohydrate, 2 Lean Protein, 3 Fat

BASIC NUTRITIONAL VALUES: **Calories** 360 | Calories from fat 190 | **Total fat** 21.0 g | Saturated fat 3.3 g | Trans fat 0.0 g | **Cholesterol** 20 mg | **Sodium** 260 mg | **Potassium** 460 mg | **Total carbohydrate** 32 g | Dietary fiber 6 g | Sugars 13 g | Added sugars 3 g | **Protein** 15 g | **Phosphorus** 345 mg

Breakfast Taco

SERVES: 1
PREP TIME: 5 minutes

SERVING SIZE: 1 taco
COOKING TIME: 5 minutes

INGREDIENTS

2 eggs
PINCH kosher salt (about 1/16 tsp)
1/8 tsp black pepper
1 tsp extra virgin olive oil
1 cup baby spinach
1 (6-inch) corn tortilla, warmed
1/4 cup canned black beans, drained and rinsed
2 Tbsp salsa
1/4 avocado

INSTRUCTIONS

1   Whisk eggs in a small bowl and season with a pinch of salt and black pepper.

2   Heat the oil in a small, nonstick pan over medium heat. Add the spinach and cook, stirring frequently, for 1 minute, or until wilted. Add the egg and cook, stirring occasionally, until egg is set, about 1 minute.

3   Remove egg from pan and place in warmed tortilla. Top with black beans, salsa, and avocado, and enjoy.

CHOICES/EXCHANGES: 1 1/2 Starch, 1/2 Carbohydrate, 2 Medium-Fat Protein, 1 1/2 Fat
BASIC NUTRITIONAL VALUES: **Calories** 370 | Calories from fat 190 | **Total fat** 21.0 g | Saturated fat 4.7 g | Trans fat 0.0 g | **Cholesterol** 370 mg | **Sodium** 520 mg | **Potassium** 770 mg | **Total carbohydrate** 30 g | Dietary fiber 9 g | Sugars 3 g | Added sugars 0 g | **Protein** 19 g | **Phosphorus** 405 mg

Simple Sweet Potato Pancakes

SERVINGS: 2

PREP TIME: 5 minutes

SERVING SIZE: 3 pancakes

COOKING TIME: 15 minutes

INGREDIENTS

1/4 cup mashed cooked sweet potato

2 large eggs

1/4 cup white whole-wheat flour (you can also use oats)

1/2 tsp baking powder

PINCH kosher salt (about 1/16 tsp)

1/2 tsp ground cinnamon

1/2 tsp chia seeds

1 tsp chopped nuts

Toppings:

1 cup sliced strawberries

2 Tbsp sugar-free syrup

INSTRUCTIONS

1   Stir the sweet potato and eggs together in a mixing bowl. Add the flour or oats along with the baking powder, salt, cinnamon, chia seeds, and nuts, and stir until combined.

2   Heat a large, nonstick skillet over medium-high heat. Drop batter 1/8 cup at a time into hot skillet. Cook until lightly browned, about 2 minutes, then flip and cook an additional 2 minutes. Repeat with remaining batter.

3   Top each serving of pancakes with 1/2 cup sliced strawberries and/or 1 Tbsp sugar-free syrup.

NOTE: *Other fruit may be substituted in place of strawberries.*

CHOICES/EXCHANGES: 1 1/2 Starch, 1/2 Fruit, 1 Medium-Fat Protein

BASIC NUTRITIONAL VALUES: **Calories** 200 | Calories from fat 50 | **Total fat** 6.0 g | Saturated fat 1.8 g | Trans fat 0.0 g | **Cholesterol** 185 mg | **Sodium** 250 mg | **Potassium** 360 mg | **Total carbohydrate** 28 g | Dietary fiber 5 g | Sugars 8 g | Added sugars 0 g | **Protein** 10 g | **Phosphorus** 315 mg

Herbed Soft Scrambled–Eggs on Toast

Adapted from: *The Clean & Simple Diabetes Cookbook*. American Diabetes Association, 2019.

SERVES: 2
PREP TIME: 5 minutes

SERVING SIZE: 1 toast
COOKING TIME: 5 minutes

Fresh herbs turn ordinary scrambled eggs into something special! Use whatever herbs you have on hand, or try any of these dynamic duos: parsley and mint, dill and chives, parsley and tarragon, or mint and basil.

For the fluffiest scrambled eggs, try gently folding rather than continuously stirring them. All you'll do is slowly scrape up beaten eggs as they cook using a flexible silicone spatula, folding (gently flopping) the cooked egg portion on top of the runnier portion. Continue just until there's no more runniness.

INGREDIENTS

1 tsp olive oil

2 eggs, beaten

1/8 tsp salt

1/4 cup loosely packed, chopped fresh herbs

2 slices sprouted whole-grain or whole-wheat bread, toasted

INSTRUCTIONS

1 Heat oil in a medium, nonstick skillet over medium-low heat. Pour the eggs into the hot skillet and cook while gently stirring (or folding) the mixture, just until the eggs are still moist but no longer runny, about 1 1/2–2 minutes. Remove the skillet from the heat, sprinkle with the salt, and gently stir (or fold) in the herbs.

2 Top each toast with half the herbed eggs. If desired, sprinkle with freshly ground black pepper to taste. Serve.

CHOICES/EXCHANGES: 1 Starch, 1 Protein, 1 Fat

BASIC NUTRITIONAL VALUES: **Calories** 170 | Calories from fat 35 | **Total fat** 8.0 g | Saturated fat 2.0 g | Trans fat 0.0 g | **Cholesterol** 185 mg | **Sodium** 290 mg | **Potassium** 190 mg | **Total carbohydrate** 16 g | Dietary fiber 3 g | Sugars 0 g | Added sugars 0 g | **Protein** 11 g | **Phosphorus** 170 mg

Salmon Toast with Greens

SERVINGS: 1
PREP TIME: 10 minutes

SERVING SIZE: 1 toast with greens
COOKING TIME: None

INGREDIENTS

1 Tbsp light cream cheese

1 slice (1 oz) sourdough or whole-grain bread, toasted

2 oz canned salmon (preferably sockeye)

1/2 tsp capers, rinsed

1/4 cup diced tomatoes

1 Tbsp finely chopped red onion

1 tsp chopped fresh dill

2 cups baby lettuce or spinach

1 Tbsp balsamic vinaigrette salad dressing

INSTRUCTIONS

1 Spread the cream cheese on toasted bread. Flake salmon and place on top of cream cheese. Garnish with capers, tomatoes, onion, and dill.

2 Toss lettuce with salad dressing and enjoy either on top of or alongside salmon toast.

CHOICES/EXCHANGES: 1 Starch, 1/2 Carbohydrate, 1 Nonstarchy Vegetable, 2 Lean Protein, 1 1/2 Fat

BASIC NUTRITIONAL VALUES: **Calories** 310 | Calories from fat 130 | **Total fat** 14.0 g | Saturated fat 3.6g | Trans fat 0.0 g | **Cholesterol** 55 mg | **Sodium** 670 mg | **Potassium** 680 mg | **Total carbohydrate** 25 g | Dietary fiber 3 g | Sugars 4 g | Added sugars 0 g | **Protein** 20 g | **Phosphorus** 290 mg

LUNCH

Bento Box

SERVINGS: 1

SERVING SIZE: 1 boxed lunch

PREP TIME: 5 minutes

COOKING TIME: None

INGREDIENTS

1/2 oz nuts (almonds, walnuts, pistachios, peanuts, etc.)

1 large hard-boiled egg

1 oz whole-grain crackers

1 cup sliced bell pepper

1/2 cup sliced cucumber

1/2 cup baby carrots

1/4 cup hummus

1/3 cup grapes

INSTRUCTIONS

1   Place ingredients in portioned bento box or other container. Enjoy at lunch!

CHOICES/EXCHANGES: 2 Starch, 1/2 Fruit, 3 Nonstarchy Vegetable, 1 Medium-Fat Protein, 3 Fat

BASIC NUTRITIONAL VALUES: **Calories** 480 | Calories from fat 210 | **Total fat** 23.0 g | Saturated fat 4.1 g | Trans fat 0.1 g | **Cholesterol** 185 mg | **Sodium** 530 mg | **Potassium** 980 mg | **Total carbohydrate** 55 g | Dietary fiber 12 g | Sugars 21 g | Added sugars 0 g | **Protein** 19 g | **Phosphorus** 430 mg

Mason Jar Salad

SERVINGS: 1
PREP TIME: 10 minutes

SERVING SIZE: 1 jar
COOKING TIME: None

INGREDIENTS

1 1/2 Tbsp Italian salad dressing

1/4 cup canned artichoke hearts, drained and rinsed

4 Kalamata olives

1/4 cup shredded carrot

1/4 cup diced red bell pepper

1/4 cup canned, no-salt-added garbanzo beans, drained and rinsed

1 hard-boiled egg, diced

1/4 cup cooked quinoa

2 Tbsp toasted, sliced, unsalted almonds

1 Tbsp crumbled feta cheese

1 1/2 cups baby lettuce or chopped romaine lettuce

INSTRUCTIONS

1 Place dressing in the bottom of a quart-size, wide-mouth jar. Top with the artichoke hearts, then the olives, carrot, bell pepper, beans, egg, quinoa, almonds, feta cheese, and lettuce. Screw on top and refrigerate until ready to eat.

2 When ready to eat, pour into a bowl and enjoy!

NOTE: *Salad can be made up to 5 days in advance.*

CHOICES/EXCHANGES: 1 1/2 Starch, 1/2 Carbohydrate, 2 Nonstarchy Vegetable, 2 Lean Protein, 4 Fat

BASIC NUTRITIONAL VALUES: **Calories** 460 | Calories from fat 230 | **Total fat** 26.0 g | Saturated fat 4.0 g | Trans fat 0.1 g | **Cholesterol** 190 mg | **Sodium** 770 mg | **Potassium** 760 mg | **Total carbohydrate** 38 g | Dietary fiber 10 g | Sugars 10 g | Added sugars 2 g | **Protein** 20 g | **Phosphorus** 395 mg

Avocado Egg Toast

SERVINGS: 1

PREP TIME: 5 minutes

SERVING SIZE: 1 toast

COOKING TIME: 5 minutes

INGREDIENTS

1 tsp extra virgin olive oil

1 large egg

PINCH kosher salt (about 1/16 tsp)

1/8 tsp black pepper

1/4 avocado, sliced

1 slice whole-grain bread, toasted

INSTRUCTIONS

1 Heat the oil in a small, nonstick skillet over medium heat. Crack the egg and add to the hot skillet. Sprinkle with salt and pepper. Cook 1 minute, then cover with a lid or piece of foil and reduce heat to low. Cook until white is set and yolk is cooked, about 4–5 minutes.

2 Smash avocado on the toast using the back of a fork. Place egg on top and serve.

NOTE: *Make your toast even more flavorful by topping with 1 tsp everything bagel seasoning, 1/8 tsp crushed red pepper, 1 Tbsp salsa, or 1 Tbsp diced vegetables, such as tomatoes, onions, or bell peppers.*

CHOICES/EXCHANGES: 1 Starch, 1 Medium-Fat Protein, 2 Fat

BASIC NUTRITIONAL VALUES: **Calories** 240 | Calories from fat 140 | **Total fat** 16.0 g | Saturated fat 3.2 g | Trans fat 0.0 g | **Cholesterol** 185 mg | **Sodium** 320 mg | **Potassium** 330 mg | **Total carbohydrate** 16 g | Dietary fiber 4 g | Sugars 2 g | Added sugars 0 g | **Protein** 11 g | **Phosphorus** 180 mg

Easy Caprese Salad

SERVINGS: 1

PREP TIME: 5 minutes

SERVING SIZE: 1 salad

COOKING TIME: None

INGREDIENTS

1 cup cherry tomatoes, halved

2 fresh basil leaves, torn

1 oz fresh mozzarella cheese, diced

PINCH kosher salt (about 1/16 tsp)

PINCH black pepper (about 1/16 tsp)

1 tsp balsamic vinegar

1/2 tsp extra virgin olive oil

INSTRUCTIONS

1 Toss tomatoes, basil, and mozzarella with salt and pepper in a bowl. Drizzle with vinegar and olive oil and enjoy.

CHOICES/EXCHANGES: 1 Nonstarchy Vegetable, 1 Medium-Fat Protein, 1/2 Fat

BASIC NUTRITIONAL VALUES: **Calories** 120 | Calories from fat 70 | **Total fat** 8.0 g | Saturated fat 3.9g | Trans fat 0.0 g | **Cholesterol** 15 mg | **Sodium** 200 mg | **Potassium** 400 mg | **Total carbohydrate** 8 g | Dietary fiber 2 g | Sugars 5 g | Added sugars 0 g | **Protein** 6 g | **Phosphorus** 140 mg

DINNER

Open-Face Turkey Burgers

SERVINGS: 4
PREP TIME: 5 minutes

SERVING SIZE: 1 burger
COOKING TIME: 10 minutes

INGREDIENTS

1 lb 93% lean ground turkey
1 Tbsp Worcestershire sauce
1/4 tsp black pepper
1/2 tsp garlic powder

For serving:
4 slices whole-wheat bread, toasted
4 large leaves romaine lettuce
4 slices ripe tomato
1 avocado, sliced

INSTRUCTIONS

1   Preheat grill to medium-high heat. Clean and lightly oil grill grates.

2   Place the turkey in a large bowl along with the Worcestershire sauce, black pepper, and garlic powder. Mix gently and shape into 4 burger patties.

3   Grill burgers 5 minutes, then flip and cook an additional 5 minutes, or until internal temperature reaches 165°F.

4   Place each burger on a slice of toast. Add the lettuce and tomato, divide the avocado evenly among the burgers, and enjoy. Add mustard, if desired.

> NOTE: *Burgers can also be prepared on the stove. Heat 1 tsp vegetable oil in a nonstick skillet (preferably cast iron) over medium heat. Add burgers and cook 5 minutes, then flip and cook an additional 5 minutes or until internal temperature reaches 165°F.*

CHOICES/EXCHANGES: 1 Starch, 4 Lean Protein, 1 1/2 Fat

BASIC NUTRITIONAL VALUES: **Calories** 320 | Calories from fat 140 | **Total fat** 15.0 g | Saturated fat 3.5 g | Trans fat 0.1 g | **Cholesterol** 85 mg | **Sodium** 260 mg | **Potassium** 640 mg | **Total carbohydrate** 18 g | Dietary fiber 5 g | Sugars 3 g | Added sugars 0 g | **Protein** 26 g | **Phosphorus** 310 mg

Sweet Potato Fries

SERVINGS: 4

PREP TIME: 10 minutes

SERVING SIZE: About 12 fries

COOKING TIME: 30 minutes

INGREDIENTS

Nonstick cooking spray

2 large (10-oz) sweet potatoes, scrubbed clean

1 Tbsp extra virgin olive oil

1/4 tsp kosher salt

1/4 tsp smoked paprika

1/4 tsp garlic powder

1/4 tsp pepper

INSTRUCTIONS

1 Preheat the oven to 425°F. Line a large, rimmed baking sheet with foil and coat liberally with nonstick cooking spray.

2 Cut the potatoes into 1/4-inch thick matchsticks. Place in a bowl along with the oil, salt, pepper, paprika, and garlic powder. Toss to coat, and spread onto prepared baking sheet.

3 Bake for 30 minutes, stirring every 10 minutes, or until golden. Enjoy.

CHOICES/EXCHANGES: 1 1/2 Starch, 1/2 Fat

BASIC NUTRITIONAL VALUES: **Calories** 130 | Calories from fat 30 | **Total fat** 3.5 g | Saturated fat 0.5 g | Trans fat 0.0 g | **Cholesterol** 0 mg | **Sodium** 160 mg | **Potassium** 550 mg | **Total carbohydrate** 24 g | Dietary fiber 4 g | Sugars 8 g | Added sugars 0 g | **Protein** 2 g | **Phosphorus** 65 mg

Chicken Chili

SERVINGS: 6
PREP TIME: 10 minutes

SERVING SIZE: About 1 1/4 cups
COOKING TIME: 35 minutes

INGREDIENTS

2 Tbsp extra virgin olive oil, divided
1 lb boneless, skinless chicken breasts,
    diced into bite-size pieces
1 small white onion, diced
1 green bell pepper, diced
2 cloves garlic, minced
1/8 tsp kosher salt
1 Tbsp chili powder
2 tsp ground cumin
1 tsp smoked paprika

1 (14.5-oz) can fire-roasted diced
    tomatoes, solids and liquid
1 (15-oz) can no-salt-added pinto beans,
    drained and rinsed
1 (4-oz) can diced green chiles
2 cups low-sodium chicken broth

Toppings:
1/4 cup + 2 Tbsp 2% plain Greek yogurt
1 avocado, diced

INSTRUCTIONS

1   Heat 1 Tbsp oil in a large pot over medium-high heat. Add the chicken and cook, stirring often, for 6–8 minutes or until chicken is browned, then remove from pot.

2   Add the remaining oil to the pot along with the onion and bell pepper. Cook until softened, about 6 minutes. Add garlic and cook 1 minute. Stir in browned chicken along with all of the spices and cook 1 more minute. Add the tomatoes, beans, green chiles, and chicken broth, and stir to combine. Bring to a boil, then reduce heat, cover partially with a lid, and simmer for 20 minutes.

3   Portion into bowls and garnish with 1 Tbsp of Greek yogurt and diced avocado.

CHOICES/EXCHANGES: 1 Starch, 1 Nonstarchy Vegetable, 3 Lean Protein, 1 Fat
BASIC NUTRITIONAL VALUES: **Calories** 290 | Calories from fat 100 | **Total fat** 11.0 g | Saturated fat 2.0 g | Trans fat 0.0 g | **Cholesterol** 45 mg | **Sodium** 470 mg | **Potassium** 800 mg | **Total carbohydrate** 23 g | Dietary fiber 8 g | Sugars 5 g | Added sugars 0 g | **Protein** 25 g | **Phosphorus** 270 mg

Baked Lemon-Mustard Sheet Pan Salmon

SERVINGS: 4

PREP TIME: 10 minutes

SERVING SIZE: 1 salmon fillet + 1 cup broccoli + 1/2 cup potatoes

COOKING TIME: 12 minutes

INGREDIENTS

2 Tbsp Dijon mustard

1 lemon, zested and juiced

2 garlic cloves, minced, divided

1 lb small red potatoes, quartered

2 Tbsp extra virgin olive oil, divided

3/4 tsp kosher salt, divided

3/4 tsp black pepper, divided

1 lb broccoli florets, cut into bite-size portions

1 lb salmon fillet, cut into 4 equal-sized portions

2 Tbsp chopped fresh parsley

INSTRUCTIONS

1 Preheat the broiler. Line a large, rimmed baking sheet with foil.

2 In a small bowl, combine the mustard, lemon juice, and garlic. Set aside.

3 Toss the potatoes in a mixing bowl with 1 Tbsp oil, 1/2 tsp salt, and 1/2 tsp black pepper. Pour mixture onto prepared pan and roast for 6 minutes. Remove from oven, stir, and push potatoes to the side.

4 Add broccoli to the pan, leaving space in the middle for the salmon, and pour remaining oil over. Place salmon pieces, skin-side down, in the middle of the baking sheet. Sprinkle salmon with 1/4 tsp salt and 1/4 tsp black pepper. Spread lemon-mustard mixture evenly over the top of each piece of salmon. Return pan to the oven and broil an additional 6–8 minutes, or until salmon is cooked through.

5 Garnish with parsley and lemon zest.

CHOICES/EXCHANGES: 1 Starch, 2 Nonstarchy Vegetable, 3 Lean Protein, 2 Fat

BASIC NUTRITIONAL VALUES: **Calories** 370 | Calories from fat 140 | **Total fat** 16.0 g | Saturated fat 2.9 g | Trans fat 0.0 g | **Cholesterol** 60 mg | **Sodium** 650 mg | **Potassium** 1,300 mg | **Total carbohydrate** 28 g | Dietary fiber 5 g | Sugars 4 g | Added sugars 0 g | **Protein** 28 g | **Phosphorus** 445 mg

Crock Pot Chicken Cacciatore

Adapted from: Diabetes Food Hub (https://www.diabetesfoodhub.org/recipes/crock-pot-chicken-cacciatore.html)

SERVES: 6

PREP TIME: 15 minutes

SERVING SIZE: 1 chicken thigh + 1 cup sauce

COOKING TIME: 4 hours

INGREDIENTS

1 onion, sliced

1 green bell pepper, seeded and sliced

2 (6-oz) cans no-salt-added tomato paste

1 (14.5-oz) can diced tomatoes

3 cloves garlic, minced

1 Tbsp Italian seasoning

6 medium (4-oz) chicken thighs, skin removed

INSTRUCTIONS

1 Place all the ingredients in a crock pot.

2 Cook on high for 4 hours.

3 Serve the chicken over whole-wheat rotini pasta, if desired.

CHOICES/EXCHANGES: 4 Nonstarchy Vegetable, 1 Lean Protein, 1/2 Fat

BASIC NUTRITIONAL VALUES: **Calories** 170 | Calories from fat 45 | **Total fat** 5.0 g | Saturated fat 1.3 g |

Trans fat 0.0 g | **Cholesterol** 70 mg | **Sodium** 200 mg | **Potassium** 930 mg | **Total carbohydrate** 18 g | Dietary fiber 4 g | Sugars 10 g | Added sugars 0 g | **Protein** 16 g | **Phosphorus** 185 mg

Grilled Salmon with Mango and Tomato Salsa

Adapted from: *Diabetes Superfoods Cookbook and Meal Planner*. American Diabetes Association, 2018.

SERVES: 6

PREP TIME: 15 minutes

SERVING SIZE: 1 salmon fillet (4 oz) + 1/2 cup salsa

COOKING TIME: 10 minutes

Mango and other fruit can add a slight sweetness to any salsa. It works particularly well with this slightly spicy salmon dish. Grilling salmon fillets with the skin on makes them easier to flip and helps prevent sticking. Oiling your grill grates can also prevent sticking: dip a balled-up paper towel in oil and rub lightly over clean grill grates.

You could also cook the salmon in the oven: Preheat oven to 425°F, and bake the salmon in a shallow baking pan for about 10 minutes, or until cooked through.

INGREDIENTS

1 Tbsp chili powder

1 Tbsp cumin

1/4 tsp garlic powder

1/4 tsp ground cinnamon

1/4 tsp salt

1 1/2 lb salmon with skin on, cut into 6 (4-oz) fillets

1 Tbsp canola oil

1 1/2 cups diced mango

1 1/2 cups diced tomatoes

1/2 cup chopped fresh cilantro

1 lemon, juiced, divided

INSTRUCTIONS

1   Preheat the grill to medium-high heat.

2   In a small bowl, combine chili powder, cumin, garlic powder, cinnamon, and salt. Sprinkle the spice mixture evenly over the salmon fillets.

3   Lightly oil the grill grates with the canola oil. Place the salmon on the grill, skin-side down. Cook uncovered for 7–8 minutes, turning halfway through. The salmon is done when it flakes easily with a fork.

4   While salmon is cooking, combine mango, tomatoes, cilantro, and half of the lemon juice in a medium bowl.

5   Remove salmon from grill and spritz with remaining lemon juice. Serve each fillet with 1/2 cup salsa.

CHOICES/EXCHANGES: 1/2 Fruit, 1 Nonstarchy Vegetable, 3 Lean Protein

BASIC NUTRITIONAL VALUES: **Calories** 220 | Calories from fat 80 | **Total fat** 9.0 g | Saturated fat 1.9 g | Trans fat 0.0 g | **Cholesterol** 60 mg | **Sodium** 190 mg | **Potassium** 640 mg | **Total carbohydrate** 10 g | Dietary fiber 2 g | Sugars 8 g | Added sugars 0 g | **Protein** 23 g | **Phosphorus** 320 mg

Cilantro Lime Quinoa

Adapted from: Diabetes Food Hub (https://www.diabetesfoodhub.org/recipes/cilantro-lime-quinoa.html)

SERVES: 6

PREP TIME: 20 minutes

SERVING SIZE: 1/2 cup

COOKING TIME: 25 minutes

Quinoa has more protein than any other grain. It is gluten-free, contains 3 g fiber per serving, and is a healthy alternative in any recipe that uses rice. Add a can of low-sodium black beans to boost the fiber and protein in this recipe.

INGREDIENTS

1 Tbsp canola oil
1 small onion, chopped
2 cloves garlic, minced
1 cup quinoa
2 cups low-sodium, fat-free chicken broth (gluten-free if needed)
2 limes, juiced, divided
1/2 cup chopped fresh cilantro

INSTRUCTIONS

1   Heat the oil in a large skillet over medium heat. Add the onions and cook for 3–4 minutes. Add the garlic and cook for 30 seconds. Reduce heat to low and add quinoa. Cook over low heat for 1–2 minutes, stirring constantly to make sure the quinoa doesn't burn.

2   Add the chicken broth and half of the lime juice, then increase the heat to medium-high and bring to a boil. Reduce heat to low, cover, and simmer for 15 minutes, or until done. Remove from heat.

3   Stir in the remaining lime juice and the cilantro, and enjoy.

CHOICES/EXCHANGES: 1 1/2 Starch, 1/2 Fat

BASIC NUTRITIONAL VALUES: **Calories** 140 | Calories from fat 35 | **Total fat** 4.0 g | Saturated fat 0.4 g | Trans fat 0.0 g | **Cholesterol** 0 mg | **Sodium** 50 mg | **Potassium** 270 mg | **Total carbohydrate** 22 g | Dietary fiber 2 g | Sugars 3 g | Added sugars 0 g | **Protein** 6 g | **Phosphorus** 160 mg

Pork Tacos

Adapted from: Diabetes Food Hub (https://www.diabetesfoodhub.org/recipes/pork-tacos.html)

SERVES: 12

PREP TIME: 45 minutes

SERVING SIZE: 1 taco

COOKING TIME: 30 minutes

This recipe calls for pork tenderloin, one of the leaner cuts of pork available. You can also top these tacos with avocado and fresh salsa.

INGREDIENTS

2 limes, juiced

2 cloves garlic, minced

1 1/2 Tbsp chili powder

1 tsp cumin

1 tsp dried oregano

1/2 tsp salt

1/2 tsp black pepper

1 1/4 lb pork tenderloin

12 low-carb, whole-wheat tortillas (10 g carb per tortilla)

2 tomatoes, diced

1 1/2 cups shredded lettuce

1 cup shredded, reduced-fat cheddar cheese

INSTRUCTIONS

1 In a large bowl combine lime juice, garlic, chili powder, cumin, oregano, salt, and pepper. Add pork and coat well. Marinate in refrigerator for 30 minutes up to 4 hours.

2 Preheat oven to 375°F. Place tenderloins in a shallow baking dish and bake for 30 minutes or until pork is done.

3 Remove pork from oven and let rest for 10 minutes. Cut pork into 1-inch chunks.

4 Serve pork in warm tortillas topped with tomatoes, lettuce, and cheese.

CHOICES/EXCHANGES: 1 Starch, 2 Lean Protein

BASIC NUTRITIONAL VALUES: **Calories** 140 | Calories from fat 50 | **Total fat** 6.0 g | Saturated fat 1.6 g | Trans fat 0.0 g | **Cholesterol** 30 mg | **Sodium** 410 mg | **Potassium** 270 mg | **Total carbohydrate** 14 g | Dietary fiber 9 g | Sugars 1 g | Added sugars 0 g | **Protein** 17 g | **Phosphorus** 190 mg

Cauliflower Fried "Rice"

Adapted from: Diabetes Food Hub (https://www.diabetesfoodhub.org/recipes/cauliflower-fried-rice.html)

SERVES: 4

PREP TIME: 15 minutes

SERVING SIZE: 1/2 cup

COOKING TIME: 13 minutes

Finely chopped cauliflower can be a remarkable nonstarchy side that's lower in calories and carbohydrate than rice. Or make it a main dish by adding chicken breast, shrimp, or tofu. To make this recipe even easier, start with packaged "riced" cauliflower that can be found fresh or frozen in many grocery stores.

INGREDIENTS

3 cups cauliflower florets

1 Tbsp olive oil, divided

2 large carrots, finely diced

3 green onions (scallions), chopped

1 tsp sesame oil

1 1/2 Tbsp reduced-sodium soy sauce

1/4 cup low-sodium, no-salt-added, fat-free chicken broth

1/8 tsp ground ginger

1/8 tsp ground black pepper

INSTRUCTIONS

1 Cut the cauliflower into small chunks and process in a food processor until florets become the size of rice, or grate the head of cauliflower with a grater. Set aside.

2 Heat 1/2 Tbsp olive oil in a nonstick pan over medium-high heat. Add carrots and green onions and sauté for 5 minutes.

3 Add remaining 1/2 Tbsp olive oil and sesame oil to pan. Add cauliflower "rice" and remaining ingredients and lower heat to medium-low. Cook for 6–8 minutes, stirring frequently, until cauliflower is tender but not mushy. Enjoy.

CHOICES/EXCHANGES: 2 Nonstarchy Vegetable, 1 Fat

BASIC NUTRITIONAL VALUES: **Calories** 80 | Calories from fat 45 | **Total fat** 5.0 g | Saturated fat 0.7 g | Trans fat 0.0 g | **Cholesterol** 0 mg | **Sodium** 260 mg | **Potassium** 530 mg | **Total carbohydrate** 8 g | Dietary fiber 3 g | Sugars 4 g | Added sugars 0 g | **Protein** 2 g | **Phosphorus** 55 mg

SNACKS & DESSERTS

Greek Yogurt Chocolate Mousse

Adapted from: *The Diabetes Cookbook*. American Diabetes Association, 2018.

SERVES: 6

PREP TIME: 10 minutes

SERVING SIZE: Heaping 1/3 cup + 1/3 cup raspberries

COOKING TIME: 1 minute

Making dessert for a special occasion? This satisfying dessert can be prepared ahead of time and refrigerated. Just before serving, portion it out and top with the whipped topping.

INGREDIENTS

6 mini Hershey's Sugar-Free Special Dark Chocolate bars, chopped

2 cups nonfat plain Greek yogurt

2 Tbsp honey or 4 packets artificial sweetener

1 tsp vanilla extract

1/4 cup skim milk

Topping:

1/4 cup + 2 Tbsp nonfat whipped topping

2 cups fresh raspberries

INSTRUCTIONS

1   Add the chopped chocolate to a microwave-safe bowl. Microwave the chocolate on high for 1 minute, then stir. If not completely melted, microwave for additional 30 seconds, then stir until all chunks are melted. If needed, repeat in 30-second cooking intervals just until the chunks are melted. Do not overcook.

2   In a medium mixing bowl, whip the Greek yogurt with an electric mixer until fluffy. Add the honey, vanilla, and milk, and beat some more. Add the melted chocolate a small amount at a time, beating in between additions.

3   Once all of the chocolate is mixed into the yogurt, divide the mousse into 6 portions and top each portion with 1/3 cup raspberries and 1 Tbsp whipped topping.

CHOICES/EXCHANGES: 1/2 Fruit, 1/2 Fat-Free Milk, 1/2 Carbohydrate, 1/2 Fat

BASIC NUTRITIONAL VALUES: **Calories** 130 | Calories from fat 35 | **Total fat** 4.0 g | Saturated fat 2.1 g | Trans fat 0.0 g | **Cholesterol** 5 mg | **Sodium** 35 mg | **Potassium** 220 mg | **Total carbohydrate** 17 g | Dietary fiber 3 g | Sugars 11 g | Added sugars 6 g | **Protein** 9 g | **Phosphorus** 145 mg

Cucumber Guacamole

Adapted from: Latin Comfort Foods Made Healthy. American Diabetes Association, 2018.

SERVES: 6   SERVING SIZE: 1/4 cup

PREP TIME: 10 minutes   COOKING TIME: None

Who doesn't love a great guac? Avocados can be enjoyed on a daily basis, but minding the serving size is key. Try to complement the avocado with a vegetable to bulk it up and reduce the amount of avocado in the recipe. Cucumber is great because it is refreshing and does not alter the flavor.

INGREDIENTS

1 Hass avocado, pitted and cubed

1 tomato, diced

1/2 seedless English cucumber (about 4 oz), finely chopped

2 Tbsp chopped fresh cilantro

1 Tbsp lime juice

1 Tbsp white wine vinegar

1/2 jalapeño pepper, minced

1/4 tsp salt

INSTRUCTIONS

1. Coarsely mash the avocado in a medium bowl. Add the tomato, cucumber, cilantro, lime juice, vinegar, jalapeño, and salt until well mixed. Serve with sliced radishes for dipping, if desired.

CHOICES/EXCHANGES: 1 Fat

BASIC NUTRITIONAL VALUES: **Calories** 45 | Calories from fat 25 | **Total fat** 3.0 g | Saturated fat 0.5 g | Trans fat 0.0 g | **Cholesterol** 0 mg | **Sodium** 100 mg | **Potassium** 200 mg | **Total carbohydrate** 4 g | Dietary fiber 2 g | Sugars 1 g | Added sugars 0 g | **Protein** 1 g | **Phosphorus** 25 mg

No-Bake Peanut Butter and Chocolate Bites

Adapted from: Diabetes Food Hub (https://www.diabetesfoodhub.org/recipes/no-bake-peanut-butter-chocolate-bites.html)

SERVES: 24

PREP TIME: 5 minutes

SERVING SIZE: 2 bites

COOKING TIME: 3 minutes

Need a healthy snack for your summer road trip? This simple treat is much better for you than any processed snack that you get at a gas station.

INGREDIENTS

1/3 cup light sugar and stevia blend
1/3 cup skim milk
1/2 cup peanut butter
1 tsp vanilla extract
2 cups rolled oats (not quick cooking)
3 Tbsp mini chocolate chips

INSTRUCTIONS

1   In a small saucepan, combine light sugar and stevia blend and milk over medium heat. Stir well and bring to a boil for 1 1/2 minutes. Stir in peanut butter and vanilla until just incorporated. Remove from heat.

2   Add oats and chocolate chips, and stir to incorporate.

3   Scoop oat mixture into 1 Tbsp balls and place on waxed paper. Let cool and refrigerate.

CHOICES/EXCHANGES: 1/2 Carbohydrate, 1 Fat

BASIC NUTRITIONAL VALUES: **Calories** 80 | Calories from fat 30 | **Total fat** 3.5 g | Saturated fat 0.7 g | Trans fat 0.0 g | **Cholesterol** 0 mg | **Sodium** 20 mg | **Potassium** 70 mg | **Total carbohydrate** 9 g | Dietary fiber 1 g | Sugars 4 g | Added sugars 3 g | **Protein** 2 g | **Phosphorus** 55 mg

Zucchini and Date Muffins

Adapted from: Diabetes Food Hub (https://www.diabetesfoodhub.org/recipes/zucchini-and-date-muffins.html)

SERVES: 12　　　　　　　　　　　**SERVING SIZE:** 1 muffin
PREP TIME: 15 minutes　　　　　　**COOKING TIME:** 30 minutes

These make a great grab-and-go breakfast for the road. You can also make this recipe into a loaf of zucchini bread if you want. Just increase the cooking time to 50–60 minutes.

INGREDIENTS

Nonstick cooking spray or 12 paper
　　muffin cups
1/3 cup Splenda Brown Sugar Blend
1/2 cup unsweetened apple sauce
1/4 cup canola oil
4 egg whites
1 tsp vanilla extract
1 cup whole-wheat flour

1 cup rolled oats
2 tsp baking powder
1 tsp baking soda
1/2 tsp salt
1 tsp ground cinnamon
1/4 cup pitted dried dates, chopped
2 cups shredded zucchini

INSTRUCTIONS

1　Preheat oven to 350°F. Lightly spray a muffin tin with nonstick cooking spray or line with paper muffin cups. Set pan aside.

2　In a medium bowl, combine Splenda Brown Sugar Blend, applesauce, oil, egg whites, and vanilla, and mix well. Set aside.

3　In a large bowl, combine flour, oats, baking powder, baking soda, salt, cinnamon, and dates. Make a well in the center of the dry ingredients, then add sugar (wet) mixture to dry ingredients all at once and mix well. Stir in zucchini.

4　Equally portion batter among the 12 muffin cups. Bake for 30 minutes or until toothpick inserted in center comes out clean.

CHOICES/EXCHANGES: 1 Starch, 1/2 Carbohydrate, 1 Fat

BASIC NUTRITIONAL VALUES: **Calories** 140 | Calories from fat 45 | **Total fat** 5.0 g | Saturated fat 0.5 g | Trans fat 0.0 g | **Cholesterol** 0 mg | **Sodium** 280 mg | **Potassium** 180 mg | **Total carbohydrate** 21 g | Dietary fiber 3 g | Sugars 6 g | Added sugars 2 g | **Protein** 4 g | **Phosphorus** 150 mg

White Bean, Lemon, and Herbed Feta Dip

Adapted from: *The Mediterranean Diabetes Cookbook, 2nd Edition*. American Diabetes Association, 2019.

SERVES: 8

PREP TIME: 15 minutes

SERVING SIZE: 1/4 cup

COOKING TIME: None

If you are a Mediterranean food fan, this dip will make a great addition to hummus in your repertoire. Note that when storing this dip in the refrigerator, it tends to firm up. Before serving, simply stir in water a tablespoon at a time until it reaches the desired consistency.

INGREDIENTS

1 1/2 cups canned or cooked cannellini beans

1/2 cup Greek feta cheese, cut into small pieces or crumbled

1 lemon, zested and juiced

1/4 cup extra virgin olive oil

1/4 cup fresh mint (plus extra for garnish)

1/4 cup fresh oregano (plus extra for garnish)

Freshly ground black pepper, to taste

INSTRUCTIONS

1   Combine cannellini beans, feta, lemon zest and juice, olive oil, mint, and oregano in a food processor. Pulsing on and off, purée until smooth.

2   Taste and season with salt (if desired) and pepper.

CHOICES/EXCHANGES: 1/2 Starch, 2 Fat

BASIC NUTRITIONAL VALUES: **Calories** 120 | Calories from fat 70 | **Total fat** 8.0 g | Saturated fat 1.9 g | Trans fat 0.1 g | **Cholesterol** 10 mg | **Sodium** 80 mg | **Potassium** 160 mg | **Total carbohydrate** 9 g | Dietary fiber 2 g | Sugars 1 g | Added sugars 0 g | **Protein** 4 g | **Phosphorus** 70 mg

Peanut Butter Banana Oat Bites

Adapted from: *The Diabetes Cookbook*. American Diabetes Association, 2018.

SERVES: 24
PREP TIME: 15 minutes

SERVING SIZE: 2 bites
COOKING TIME: 11 minutes

These satisfying high-fiber bites make a great snack or quick breakfast. You can freeze a couple bites in a snack-size plastic bag for a grab-and-go breakfast, too!

INGREDIENTS

1/2 cup peanut butter

1 ripe banana, mashed

1 egg

1 tsp vanilla extract

2 Tbsp Splenda Brown Sugar Blend

2 cups rolled oats (not quick cooking; gluten-free if needed)

1 tsp baking soda

1/2 tsp salt

1/4 cup ground flaxseed

INSTRUCTIONS

1   Preheat oven to 350°F. Line a baking sheet with parchment paper.

2   Heat peanut butter in microwave for 30 seconds. Transfer to a medium bowl and whisk together with banana, egg, vanilla, and Splenda Brown Sugar Blend.

3   In a small bowl, mix together oats, baking soda, salt, and ground flaxseed. Add oat mixture to peanut butter mixture and mix well.

4   Scoop batter into 1 Tbsp balls and place on baking sheet. Bake for 10–12 minutes. Cool on wire rack.

CHOICES/EXCHANGES: 1/2 Carbohydrate, 1 Fat

BASIC NUTRITIONAL VALUES: **Calories** 70 | Calories from fat 35 | **Total fat** 4.0 g | Saturated fat 0.8 g | Trans fat 0.0 g | **Cholesterol** 10 mg | **Sodium** 130 mg | **Potassium** 90 mg | **Total carbohydrate** 8 g | Dietary fiber 1 g | Sugars 2 g | Added sugars 1 g | **Protein** 3 g | **Phosphorus** 60 mg

Chunky Pistachio Granola

SERVES: 9

PREP TIME: 15 minutes

SERVING SIZE: About 1/2 cup

COOKING TIME: 30 minutes

INGREDIENTS

3 1/2 cups rolled oats

1 cup lightly salted pistachios, chopped

1 tsp ground cinnamon

1/8 tsp kosher salt

2 Tbsp flax seeds

2 Tbsp avocado oil (or other neutral-flavored oil)

2 Tbsp coconut oil

3 Tbsp honey

1 large egg white, lightly beaten

INSTRUCTIONS

1 Preheat oven to 325°F. Line a jelly roll pan with parchment paper.

2 In a large mixing bowl, combine oats, pistachios, cinnamon, salt, and flax seeds. Set aside.

3 In a small, microwave-safe bowl, combine the avocado oil, coconut oil, and honey. Microwave on high for 20-second intervals, stirring after each interval, until melted.

4 Pour oil mixture over oat mixture. Using a silicone spatula, toss and turn to coat oat mixture evenly. Add the egg white and stir to combine.

5 Spread mixture evenly onto prepared pan and push down onto pan. Bake for 30 minutes, rotating pan once halfway through cooking time, then transfer pan to a wire rack to cool.

6 Once cool, break into clusters. Store in an air-tight container. Enjoy within 1 week.

CHOICES/EXCHANGES: 1 1/2 Starch, 1/2 Carbohydrate, 2 1/2 Fat

BASIC NUTRITIONAL VALUES: **Calories** 185 | Calories from fat 100 | **Total fat** 11 g | Saturated fat 2.8 g | Trans fat 0.0 g | **Cholesterol** 0 mg | **Sodium** 45 mg | **Potassium** 190 mg | **Total carbohydrate** 22 g | Dietary fiber 4 g | Sugars 5 g | Added sugars 4 g | **Protein** 5 g | **Phosphorus** 140 mg

Dark Chocolate–Covered Strawberries

SERVES: 1
PREP TIME: 5 minutes

SERVING SIZE: 5 strawberries
COOKING TIME: 2 minutes

INGREDIENTS

1/2 oz 60%–70% dark chocolate (about 1 square), broken into small chunks
5 whole strawberries, washed and dried
1 Tbsp pistachios (without shells), finely chopped

INSTRUCTIONS

1 Heat chocolate chunks in microwavable bowl for 1 minute. Remove, stir, and place in microwave for another 30–45 seconds until chocolate is melted and smooth.

2 Line a plate or baking sheet with parchment paper and set aside. Place chopped pistachios in a small bowl.

3 Dip a strawberry into melted chocolate, then into chopped pistachios. Set strawberry on the prepared plate or baking sheet.

4 Repeat step 3 with the remaining strawberries.

5 Refrigerate for 20 minutes or until chocolate is hardened. Enjoy!

CHOICES/EXCHANGES: 1 carb, 2 fat

BASIC NUTRITIONAL VALUES: **Calories** 140 | Calories from fat 81 | **Total fat** 9.0 g | Saturated fat 3.5 g | Trans fat 0 g | **Cholesterol** 0 mg | **Sodium** 0 mg | **Potassium** 163 mg | **Total carbohydrate** 14 g | Dietary fiber 3 g | Sugars 8 g | Added sugars 4 g | **Protein** 3 g | **Phosphorus** 50 mg

MANAGING STRESS

*"I was prepared for the physical aspect of diabetes,
but not the mental toll it could take, or the isolation
I felt at times. I wish I had known about peer support
during pregnancy and that I could find other women
who shared my concerns and anxieties."*

—Ana Norton, diabetes advocate and founder & CEO of Diabetes Sisters,
lives with type 1 diabetes and is a mom of a healthy boy.

In my 19 years living with diabetes, pregnancy has been one of the hardest challenges I had to face—physically, due to the constant changes my body had to go through, but also emotionally. The combination of hormones plus the stress of managing a 24/7 chronic condition made it unbearable at times. But the journey and the end result—two healthy and beautify baby girls—were all worth it. Managing a chronic condition like diabetes requires two brains: a normal brain and a diabetes brain. The diabetes brain is busy thinking of what foods to eat, how much insulin to take, when to check blood glucose, and so on. At times it becomes hard to maintain both.

This chapter will discuss the real-life psychological aspects of managing diabetes in pregnancy as well as tips to stay "sane" during those 9 months. It will cover resources like support groups, discuss ways your partner/family can help, and provide relaxation techniques to stay healthy, happy, and relaxed during pregnancy.

Stress Can Affect Your Diabetes

Diabetes management can wear you out. In fact, diabetes burnout is a prevalent condition among people with diabetes. Diabetes burnout refers to a mental state in which people with diabetes feel overwhelmed, frustrated, angry, and isolated, and at times feel controlled by their diabetes. For pregnant women with diabetes, the additional burden of being responsible for a tiny human can create a lot of potential for stress!

When people with diabetes experience physical or emotional stress, their blood glucose rises. This is partly due to the fight or flight response. When you are stressed, your body releases hormones called adrenaline and cortisol, which increase insulin resistance and elevate blood glucose levels as a result. Being constantly stressed during your pregnancy will make it harder to manage your blood glucose. Although it's impossible to eliminate all the stress in our lives, there are several ways to reduce it (Table 29.1).

TABLE 29.1 Examples of Ways to Reduce Everyday Stress

Source of stress	Ways to reduce it
Long drive to work	• Listen to a podcast • Use a relaxation app
Don't have time to cook	• Meal prep on weekends • Talk to your family/partner
Blood glucose is always high at night	• Keep close logs of blood glucose and food eaten • Talk to your diabetes educator on how to improve this
Gaining too much weight	• Take a quick walk after lunch or dinner
Can't eat what you want	• Meet with a registered dietitian • Find the carbs and nutrition label of that favorite food to see if you can add it to your meal plan

Manage Your Expectations

Perfection is not the goal; your goal should be attainable and realistic. The feeling of guilt is inevitable when you live with diabetes and are expecting. You feel guilty for having a higher blood glucose value, which can lead to feeling as though you are a bad person simply because you have a blood glucose of 200 mg/dL. On top of this, you are hormonal and feel entirely responsible for your baby.

Remember that many factors affect your blood glucose, especially during pregnancy, and not all of them are under your control (e.g., pregnancy hormones). There are no "good" or "bad" numbers, just as you are not a bad person because you have a high blood glucose value. The important lesson is to learn healthy coping skills and set realistic expectations during this stressful time. Take small steps and realize where the source of your stress is coming from. Once you identify the problem, it's easier to formulate a solution with the help of your diabetes team and loved ones.

"Social support is so important. Talk to other women who have gone through pregnancy with type 1 diabetes. Also, make sure your partner understands the basics and realizes your diabetes management will need to change throughout pregnancy. You will need a shoulder to lean on!"

—Jennifer Smith, RD, LD, CDCES, Director of Lifestyle and Nutrition at Integrated Diabetes Services. She has lived with type 1 diabetes for 32 years, is co-author of a book on pregnancy with type 1 diabetes, and is a mom of two healthy kids.

Strategies to Stay Sane During Pregnancy

- **Exercise** — Exercise will be one of the most effective strategies to help you unwind. Additionally, it will provide you with some other perks, like lowering blood glucose. Even a short

10–15 minute walk will clear your mood and brain. You get a bang for your buck!

- **Keep a journal**—For some people, writing can be a sort of therapy. Focus on the things you are grateful for, but don't be afraid to vent your frustrations.
- **Be kind to yourself**—Have realistic expectations and don't beat yourself up for what you can't control. Diabetes management is not about being perfect.
- **Be positive**—It's hard not to get sidetracked by the daily frustrations, so try to focus on the ultimate goal: having a healthy baby. This is all worth it!
- **Let other people know how they can help you**—Many times, the people that most care about you want to help, but they don't know how. It's not because they don't care; it's just tough for them to understand what you are going through. That said, tell them how you are feeling and what they can do to help. Whether it's as simple as providing encouragement, not buying certain types of food, or joining you for a walk, the more specific you can be, the better your friends and family can support you.
- **Look for online support groups**—Diabetes is a 24/7 condition that can often leave you feeling lonely. Knowing someone that lives with diabetes and empathizes with your issues can be life-changing. Online diabetes communities serve as a safe space where people can connect and share similar experiences. Make sure you find communities with trustworthy information.
- **Talk to someone**—Don't be afraid to seek the help of a skilled professional, such as a therapist. A psychologist or therapist can teach you coping skills that will help you manage the daily struggles involved in diabetes care.
- **Be social and make time for friends**—Your friends and family will be the biggest source of support. Lean on them for support and even for good laughing therapy.

Resources

Realize you are not alone. Many, many women have had successful pregnancies while managing diabetes. The online diabetes community can be a great resource to connect with people who are going through similar experiences. Because as much as your family and/or partner support you, there is an innate connection among people who have truly lived it. Below are some great resources and online communities that can provide helpful tips. Just remember, everyone is different, and there are no two lives with diabetes that are alike. Make sure to talk to your diabetes healthcare team before considering any changes in your diabetes care.

Resources and Online Communities
For more, visit goodlifediabetes.com/communities

- American Diabetes Association: diabetes.org/resources
- GoodLifediabetes: goodlifediabetes.com/pregnancyand diabetes
- DiabetesSisters: diabetessisters.org
- Beyond Type 1: beyondtype1.org
- Diabetes Strong: diabetesstrong.com
- EsTuDiabetes: estudiabetes.org
- Diabetes Food Hub: diabetesfoodhub.org

Stress & Mindful Meditation Apps
- Grateful
- Happify
- iSleepeasy
- Insight Timer
- Headspace
- Calm

chapter 30

Q&A AND
DEBUNKING MYTHS

For more Q&A, visit
goodlifediabetes.com

- **If I have type 1 diabetes, will my baby have diabetes?**
  Not necessarily. The genetic risk factors associated with type 1
  diabetes are not well understood. Genes play a role, but
  researchers have also noted that factors such as environment,
  race, geography, weather, nutrition, and other autoimmune
  conditions are involved. If you are older than 25 and have
  type 1 diabetes, the chances your baby will develop diabetes
  are 1%. In the case of the general population (with no
  parents with type 1 diabetes), the risk is 0.3%. If you are
  younger than 25 years, the risk increases to about 4%. Interestingly, if the father has type 1 diabetes, the risk goes up to
  6%, and if you were diagnosed younger than 11 years of age,
  then the risk doubles. Finally, if both parents have diabetes,

the risk is not entirely known but it is expected to be even higher.[1]

● **If I have type 2 diabetes or gestational diabetes, will my baby have diabetes?**

In the case of type 2 diabetes, there is a stronger link to family history and genetics than type 1. The risk of children developing diabetes later in life is around 14%. However, we also know that environment, lifestyle, and healthy habits in early childhood also play a role. With gestational diabetes, the risk of your baby developing diabetes is similar to that of women with type 2 diabetes. Even though the risk of developing diabetes is higher than women without diabetes, it should not discourage you from pregnancy.

● **Do I need to eliminate all carbs from my diet?**

No. Carbohydrates are an essential food group that provides you and your baby energy, not to mention important nutrients like fiber, B vitamins, and folic acid. Because carbs turn into glucose, they impact your blood glucose the most. You will likely need to be more consistent in monitoring carbohydrate intake and pay close attention to how much, what type, and when to eat carbs. Remember, the best way to know if your meal plan is working is your blood glucose levels. (Make sure to also read: chapter 3, "What Can I Eat with Gestational Diabetes"; chapter 10, "Everything You Need to Know about Nutrition and Type 2 Diabetes"; and chapter 16, "Strategies to Avoid Spikes in Blood Glucose".)

● **Will insulin harm my baby?**

Absolutely not! Insulin is the preferred medication because it will not cross the placenta. Furthermore, insulin has the longest track record because it's been studied the most in treating women with diabetes during pregnancy. In fact, insulin will help your body assimilate carbohydrates much better. If you are not currently used to taking insulin, it can be very scary, but taking insulin does not mean you have failed. Insulin will prevent you from having higher blood glucose and thus prevent unnecessary complications for you and your baby, such as preeclampsia, a larger baby, and more. In the case of women with type 1 diabetes, without insulin, we would not survive.

- **Can I inject insulin in my stomach?**
The best place to give an insulin injection is where there is more fatty tissue. Sites can include arms, stomach, and upper and outer buttocks. Yes, I know it can feel strange to take insulin in your stomach, but no worries, it will not be harmful to your baby. The injection will not cross the muscle or hurt your baby. You want to keep 2 inches away from the belly button and rotate the injection sites constantly so you don't develop lumps.

- **Can I eat sugar?**
Sugar is a type of carbohydrate that can be found in both natural sources, like fruits (fructose) and milk/yogurt (lactose), in addition to added sugars. You want to try to limit the sources of added sugar, such as sweetened beverages, syrups, agave, and regular table sugar, since they provide limited nutrition. However, this doesn't mean you can't indulge in an occasional treat as long as you are aware of the total carbohydrates and include them in your meal plan. For example, 1/2 cup of regular ice cream might have 15 g of total carbohydrate, the same carbohydrate as a slice of bread. This doesn't mean they are equal nutritionally, but they do contain similar carbs, and if you are using insulin, you will take the appropriate dose based on the total grams.

- **I heard I should avoid fruits at night and in the morning. Is this true?**
There is limited evidence to show that eating fruits at night or in the morning versus another time of day will cause a

considerable rise in blood glucose. However, anecdotally, as women enter the last trimester of pregnancy they are more resistant to insulin and find they need to eat smaller amounts of carbohydrates. Fruits can be harder to manage in the morning if you are seeing a greater resistance at this time. Furthermore, you might find certain fruits with a higher glycemic index harder to manage during pregnancy. A helpful strategy is to save your fruit for lunch or dinner instead. Fruits provide an important source of fiber, water, vitamin C, and potassium. They do contain carbohydrates, so you need to be aware of the recommended portion size and total carbohydrates if you are counting carbs and matching insulin. But you should not be afraid of fruits or eliminate them.

- **Will I need to have a C-section?**
No, being pregnant and having diabetes does not mean you will need to have a C-section. The time your baby arrives is based on many things, including the size of your baby, your medical team, the presence of complications, and individual preferences. Women with uncomplicated pregnancies can safely deliver at full term (39–40 weeks). Others may have a scheduled C-section at 38 weeks. Don't feel guilty if you need to have a C-section. The important thing is to focus on delivering a healthy baby.

- **Do I need to keep insulin refrigerated at all times?**
Once you open a vial or insulin pen, you do not need to keep it refrigerated. Insulin can be stored at room temperature for 28 days. The unused insulin should be kept in the refrigerator until it's ready to open. Avoid very hot or humid places.

- **Can I breastfeed if I have diabetes?**
Absolutely! In fact, breastfeeding your baby boosts immunity, is associated with a lower risk of diabetes and autoimmune diseases, and decreases the risk of allergies. Women with preexisting diabetes are at increased risk for lactation complications like mastitis, reduced milk production, and

candida infections compared to women who don't have diabetes. Make sure to read the breastfeeding tips in chapters 6, 13, and 22.

- **Are sugar-free products better for my diabetes?**
Not necessarily. Remember, sugar-free does not mean carbohydrate-free or calorie-free. A sugar-free cookie, for example, still contains carbohydrates from the flour or even chocolate. But it can contain a lower amount of carbs because the sugar is replaced with an artificial sweetener. Your best bet is to read the label and evaluate what makes better sense. Keep in mind, eating too many sugar-free products can upset your stomach due to the sugar alcohols.

- **I had a few 200–300 mg/dL blood glucose readings in the first trimester of pregnancy. Will this harm my baby?**
One or two high blood glucose values will probably not be the deciding factor, but rather persistent elevated blood glucose. It is true that the first trimester is critical in your baby's organ development. Maintaining tight blood glucose control during this period is essential in avoiding complications. But try to focus on the whole and not on just one or two readings. If you need help managing your blood glucose, make sure you discuss these concerns with your team.

- **Can I follow a keto diet in pregnancy?**
According to the research and healthcare experts, going keto during pregnancy is not safe or recommended. Research studies done in mice with mothers following a ketogenic diet showed problems with mice offspring, including stunted growth, organ dysfunction, and smaller hearts. Even though there are limited studies, eliminating an entire food group can put your baby at risk for significant nutritional deficiencies and growth problems. The popular ketogenic diet is based on eliminating all carbohydrates and eating a very high-fat diet with moderate protein. The traditional keto diet is comprised

of 75% calories coming from fat, 20% from protein, and only 5% from carbohydrate. The ultimate goal of this trendy diet is to be in a state of ketosis. Ketosis occurs when ketones are generated due to the elimination of carbs and an increase in fats. In people with type 1 diabetes, moderate to high ketones can lead to diabetic ketoacidosis (DKA)—a very dangerous condition that requires hospitalization. Some studies have shown ketones in pregnancy is associated with adverse effects. Excess ketones can affect your baby's IQ, so we want to get rid of them as quickly as possible

- **If I am overweight and pregnant, should I focus on losing weight?**

No, pregnancy is not the time to lose weight or go on restrictive diets. It will be important to make sure to include a healthy, balanced meal plan that provides essential nutrients for your baby to grow. Instead, you should focus on maintaining a healthy weight and avoiding gaining too much weight. Read chapter 4 "Maintaining a Healthy Weight and Staying Active During Pregnancy," and chapter 12, "Exercise and Staying Active."

- **If I have gestational diabetes during pregnancy, will I always have diabetes? Or will it go away after?**

The good news is that, in most cases, gestational diabetes goes away almost immediately after giving birth. But keep in mind you are at a higher risk of developing type 2 diabetes later in life in addition to having gestational diabetes in your following pregnancies. (There is a 50% chance of developing gestational diabetes in future pregnancies,[2] and and estimated lifetime risk of up to 70% for developing type 2 diabetes.[3]) You can minimize this risk by maintaining a healthy weight, staying active, and eating a wholesome, nutritious diet. (Make sure to read chapter 6, "Delivery and the Future Ahead in Gestational Diabetes.")

REFERENCES

[1] Learn the genetics of diabetes [Internet], c2020. Arlington, VA, American Diabetes Association. Available from https://www.diabetes.org/diabetes/genetics-diabetes

[2] Schwartz N, Nachum Z, Green MS. The prevalence of gestational diabetes mellitus recurrence—effect of ethnicity and parity: a metaanalysis. *Am J Obstet Gynecol* 2015;213(3):310–317

[3] Kim C, Newton KM, Knopp RH. Gestational diabetes and the incidence of type 2 diabetes: a systematic review. *Diabetes Care* 2002;25(10):1862–1868

CHAPTER 31

WHEN TO CALL
A DOCTOR

opefully you won't experience any of these symptoms, but it's good to keep an eye on the following and learn what to do before it can become something more serious.

- **Ketones present**—Ketones are the waste products created when there is not enough insulin in the system. In gestational diabetes, ketones can appear if there is not enough carbohydrate or energy consumed. Usually, your body uses sugar (glucose) for energy, but when there is not enough glucose or insulin available, the body breaks down fat into energy, which produces ketones. In people with type 1 diabetes, moderate to high ketones can lead to DKA—a very dangerous condition that requires hospitalization. Some studies have shown ketones in pregnancy are associated with adverse effects. Excess ketones can affect your baby's IQ, so we want to get rid of them as quickly as possible. For more information on ketones and low-carb diets, please see chapter 2, "Managing Blood Glucose."

- **Fever**—Anytime you run a fever, you want to notify your doctor. Having a fever can be a sign of an infection, but it will be important to understand the root cause. Speak to your doctor as to which medications are safe to take to lower the fever, such as acetaminophen.

- **Persistent hypoglycemia**—Having persistent hypoglycemia can be very dangerous for you and your baby. If you are having trouble keeping down food and, therefore, can't drink juice or gel, then you should call your doctor right away. Hypoglycemia can cause you to lose consciousness and potentially harm your baby. Make sure to have glucagon readily available.

- **Severe or persistent vomiting/diarrhea**—If you are vomiting persistently due to morning sickness and are therefore having consistent low blood glucose that you can't correct, you need to call your doctor. Vomiting and diarrhea place you at a high risk of dehydration, which can trigger labor. You might need medication to stop the vomiting and make sure you are adequately hydrated.

- **Constant high blood glucose or low blood glucose for more than 2–3 days**—If you are noticing blood glucose out of range, this is probably a sign you need an adjustment in insulin dosage. You and your healthcare team might feel comfortable with you making self-adjustments, but if not, make sure you speak to your doctor or diabetes educator to assist you in making the necessary changes. For more guidance on insulin adjustments, make sure to read section 3, "Type 1 Diabetes and Pregnancy."

APPS AND BEST
TOOLS TO USE

Having diabetes means being on top of a lot of things. Fortunately, there is an app for that! Many different apps are
available to help you ease the burden of carb counting, medications, de-stressing, record keeping, and more. Below are some of
my favorites.

Nutrition Apps
- CalorieKing
- MyFitnessPal
- MyPlate
- Fooducate
- Figwee

Websites
- American Diabetes Association (diabetes.org)
- Beyond Type 1 (beyondtype1.com)
- Diabetes Strong (diabetesstrong.com)
- GoodlifeDiabetes (goodlifediabetes.com)
- Academy of Nutrition and Dietetics (eatright.org)
- Taking Control of Your Diabetes (tcoyd.org)
- DiabetesSisters (diabetessisters.org)
- Diatribe (diatribe.org)

Stress Management Apps
- Grateful
- Happify
- iSleepeasy
- Insight Timer
- Headspace
- Calm

Medication Management
- InPen
- Insulin Calculate

Record Keeping/Logging
- MySugr

Online Diabetes Peer Support
- Diatribe
- Beyond Type 1
- Beyond Type 2
- Diabetes Sisters
- Diabetes Strong
- Tu Diabetes
- Diabetes Self-Management
- Type 1 Nation
- Glu
- Diabetes Mine

FOOD SAFETY

Food safety is important for everyone, but it's especially important in pregnant women. Pregnant women run a higher risk of foodborne illness due to a weakened immune system. It will be important for you to practice safe food handling and know which foods to avoid as they can pose a significant risk to your baby, especially in the first trimester.

The most common food contaminants or food germs include:

- **Listeria (Listeria monocytogens)** — Very dangerous infection that can cause serious risk to you and your baby. Capable of growing in refrigerated and ready-to-eat foods like meats, hot dogs, and unpasteurized dairy.

- **T. Gondii (Toxoplasma gondii)** — Can cause toxoplasmosis, a dangerous condition that can cross the placenta and harm your baby. Primary sources include raw or undercooked meats, unwashed fruits, and veggies.
- **E. Coli (Escherichia coli)** — Can be found in undercooked or raw beef, unpasteurized raw milk, and juices. Usually causes diarrhea and abdominal cramps.
- **Salmonella** — Mostly found in undercooked proteins like eggs, meat, fish, or raw dairy or unpasteurized juices. Symptoms include abdominal pain, diarrhea, dehydration.

Below are some simple steps you can take to prevent contamination and stay safe:

1. **Clean** — Always wash your hands before handling food. Sounds basic, I know. Make sure you rinse raw fruits and veggies. Clean cutting boards, dishes, utensils, and countertops with hot water and soap.
2. **Separate** — Separate raw produce such as meat, seafood, and eggs from ready-to-eat foods. Make sure you have separate cutting boards for raw meats and another for produce.
3. **Cook Properly** — Cooking destroys harmful bacteria. Keep food out of the danger zone where bacteria love to thrive: 40°F–140°F. Make sure you discard food that is left out at room temperature for more than 2 hours.

Find more information and an FAQ at the FDA's Food Safety for moms to be: fda.gov/food/people-risk-foodborne-illness/food-safety-moms-be

INDEX

Note: Page numbers followed by *t* refer to tables. Page numbers in **bold** indicate an in-depth discussion.

A

A1C
blood glucose target, 14–15, 89–90, 156*t*
continuous glucose monitor, 92, 178–179
first trimester, 184, 189
gestational diabetes, 70
insulin pump, 174
preconception planning, 87–88, 153–154, 161
type 1 diabetes, 155
abortion, spontaneous, 80
Academy of Nutrition and Dietetics, 110, 336
ACE inhibitor. *See* angiotensin-converting enzyme (ACE) inhibitors

acetaminophen, 334
added sugar, 247
adrenaline, 187, 320
aerobic exercise, 137–138
African American population, 8
agave nectar, 254, 289, 293
allergic conditions, 68, 69*t*, 145, 216, 232, 328
American College of Obstetricians and Gynecologists (ACOG), 52, 63, 66, 67*t*, 137, 145, 207, 215
American Diabetes Association (ADA), 155, 323, 336
Complete Guide to Carb Counting, 122
Standards of Medical Care in Diabetes, 14, 89
amino acid, 32

heart disease, 35, 95, 184
heart problems, 154
hemoglobin A1c. *See* A1C
herb, 296, 315
Herbed Soft Scrambled Eggs on Toast,
265–266, 268
Herbed Soft Scrambled Eggs on Toast, 296
high blood glucose
birth defect, 154
constant, 334
continuous glucose monitor, 17,
91–92
diabetes defined, 6
exercise, 139*t*
first trimester, 329
insulin duration, 197
ketone, 23
labor and delivery, 206–207
postdelivery, 67
prenatal education visit, 88, 157
reasons and solutions, 20–21
second trimester, 194
symptoms, 139*t*
type 2 diabetes, 78
high blood pressure, 62, 94–96, 107,
139, 184, 232, 248
high-risk pregnancy, 85
honeydew melon, 290
hormone
blood glucose, 20
contra-insulin, 200
exercise, 52
first trimester, 184, 187
high blood glucose, 59–60
insulin, 7, 167
insulin pump, 174, 175*t*
insulin resistance, 43, 79, 117
insulin-to-carb ratio, 176
labor and delivery, 142
meal timing, 169
morning sickness, 240
postdelivery, 215
pregnancy, 7, 60, 79, 169, 174, 193,
196–197, 200
second trimester, 193–194, 196
stress, 321

human placental hormone, 192, 196
hummus
fat, 251*t*
lunch, 256, 258, 260, 298
snack, 252, 274–277, 279, 281–282,
284, 286, 288
hunger, 192
hybrid closed-loop pump, 180
hydration, 241–242
hyperemesis, 240
hyperglycemia. *See* high blood glucose
hypertension. *See* high blood pressure
hypoglycemia. *See* low blood glucose
hypoglycemia unawareness, 17, 87,
155, 184–187

I

immune system, 68–69, 145, 216
immunization, 162
infection, 69*t*, 145*t*, 146, 334, 337
ingredient, 248
injection, 93–94
InPen, 336
Insight Timer, 323, 336
Institute of Medicine, 112
insulin
adjustment, 334
aspart, 61, 104*t*, 105
basal, 104*t*, 105–106, 175*t*
basal rate, 174, 176, 186, 188, 192,
196–197, 209, 217
blood glucose checking, 18
blood glucose level, 60–61
bolus, 104*t*, 105, 166–167, 170, 174,
175*t*, 176–177, 180, 196–197
C-section, 68
degludec, 61, 104*t*, 106
detemir, 61, 104*t*, 106
dosage, 42
dual-wave bolus, 177, 197, 201
duration, 177, 197
exercise, 52–53, 139
extended bolus, 177
first trimester, 184–186
fourth trimester, 215